WP LIFE SERIES

Super Healthy
Pregnancy
Supercharged

Lisa Guy N.D.

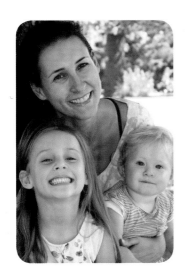

Lisa Guy is a highly qualified naturopath, author, and passionate foodie with over a decade of clinical experience. Lisa runs a busy Sydney based clinic called Art of Healing. Lisa has a real love for helping people achieve true health and happiness, through good wholesome foods, nutritional supplementation, healing herbs and homeopathic remedies. Lisa is an avid health writer, regularly writing for a number of top newspapers, magazines, and health and natural parenting websites. Lisa is the author of *My Goodness: all you need to know about children's health and nutrition*, *Heal Yourself*, *Pregnancy Essentials*, and *Listen to Your Body*.

Lisa Guy, ND

Adv ND, Adv Herb Med, Adv Hom, Adv Nut, BHSc.
www.artofhealing.com.au
www.facebook.com/ArtOfHealingNaturopathicMedicine
www.instagram.com/lisaguy_artofhealing

For my two gorgeous girls, Lily and Sienna.

Published by
Wilkinson Publishing Pty Ltd
ACN 006 042 173
Level 4, 2 Collins Street, Melbourne, Vic 3000
Tel: 03 9654 5446 www.wilkinsonpublishing.com.au

National Library of Australia Cataloguing-in-Publication entry

Author:	Guy, Lisa, author.
Title:	Super healthy pregnancy supercharged / Lisa Guy.
ISBN:	9781922178596 (paperback)
Series:	WP life series.
Subjects:	Pregnancy--Nutritional aspects Pregnancy--Health aspects. Prenatal care. Cooking.
Dewey Number:	618.242

International distribution by Pineapple Media Ltd
(www.pineapple-media.com) Photos by agreement with Getty/Thinkstock.
Recipe photography by agreement with Lisa Guy.
Design by Joanna Hunt
Printed in China

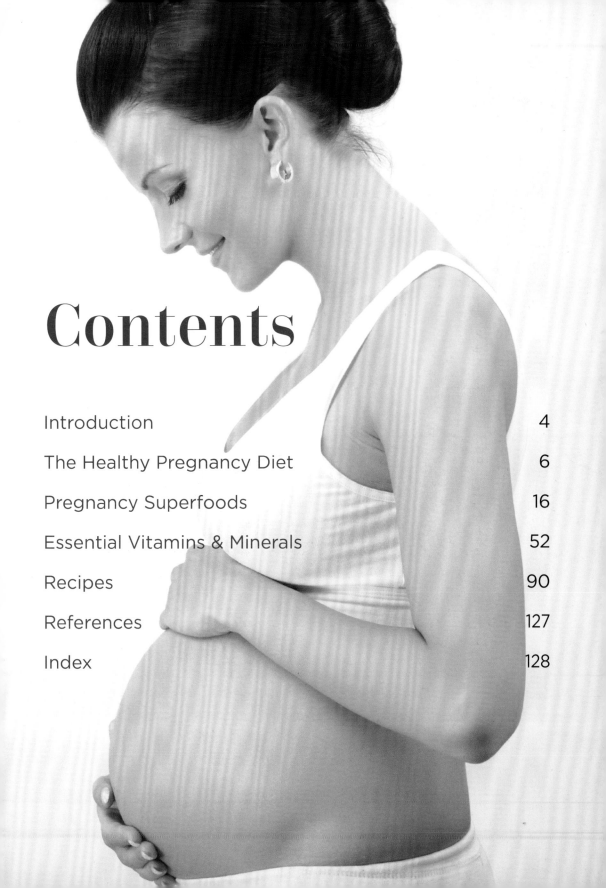

Contents

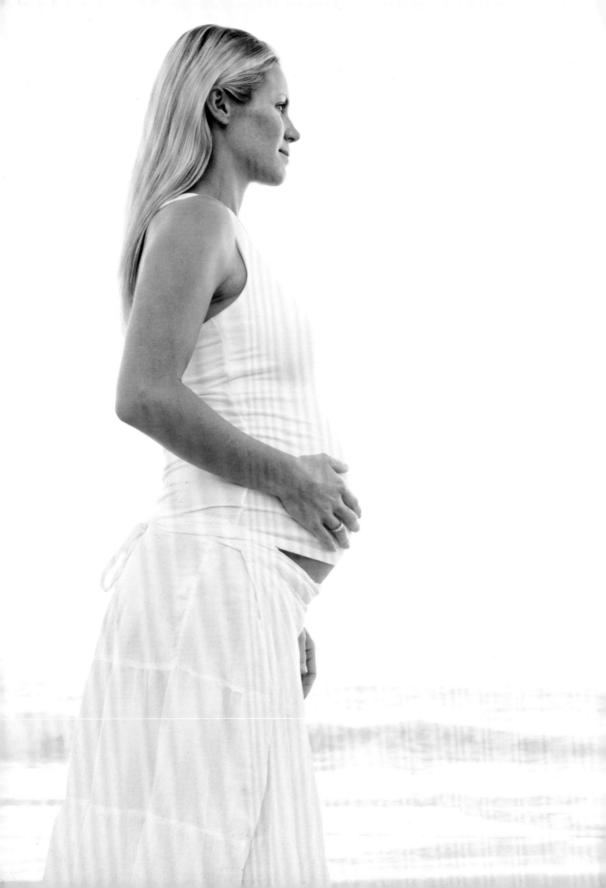

Introduction

Congratulations on your incredible news! Let me tell you that you're about to embark on one of the greatest journeys of your life.

Being pregnant is an exciting and important time. There is such wonder and joy at every turn, and of course a little apprehension as well.

Forty weeks of pregnancy may seem long at first, but believe me it goes extremely quickly. So you want to try to slow down and enjoy it as much as you can. You are about to go through many profound physical and psychological changes as those pregnancy hormones start racing around your body. Of course there's also the growth of a big, gorgeous belly, and those extra lovely womanly curves, which you should embrace with vigor. Pregnancy is a truly amazing ride, so try to enjoy every moment!

Over the next 40 weeks, you have the very important task of nourishing and supporting the growth and development of your little one. Your diet and health habits during pregnancy, and later when breastfeeding, have a direct impact on your baby's health, now and later in life. Small wonder mums-to-be are bombarded with so much health information from both the media and well-meaning family and friends. It can all get very overwhelming and confusing!

Over the last 12 years as a naturopath and nutritionist, I've experienced the genuine thrill of supporting countless women on their journeys through pregnancy and beyond. I have been lucky enough to have given birth to two beautiful little girls myself. So through my research, and clinical and personal experience, I've put together this wonderful resource book, *Super Healthy Pregnancy Supercharged*. This book contains everything expectant mums need to know about how best to nourish themselves and their growing babies, so as to have the best pregnancy and healthiest baby possible. This book will show mums-to-be how to supercharge their diet with a variety of pregnancy super foods, optimising their health and that of their baby's. Along with plenty of practical nutritional advice and tips for preventing common pregnancy ailments such as constipation, anaemia and morning sickness.

Wishing you love and best wishes for a wonderful pregnancy and a super healthy baby,

Lisa

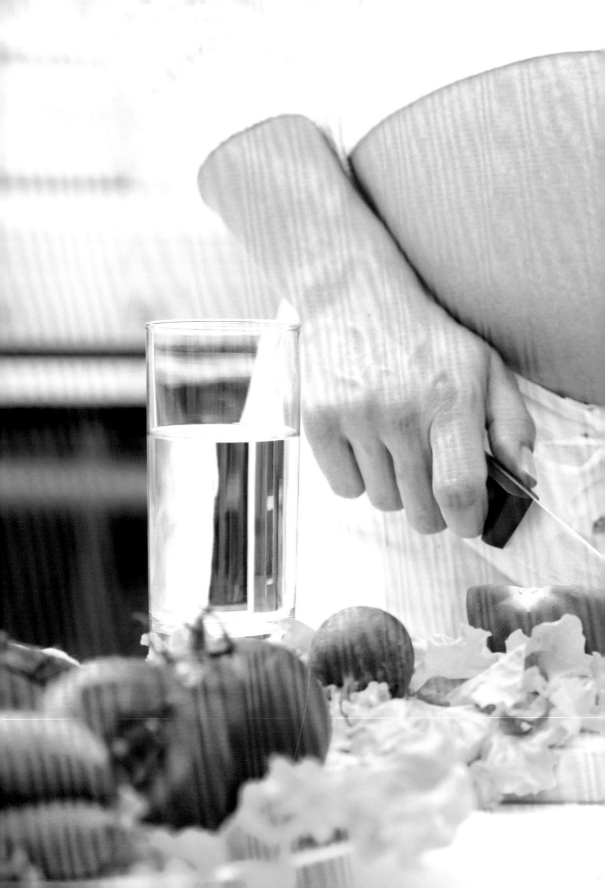

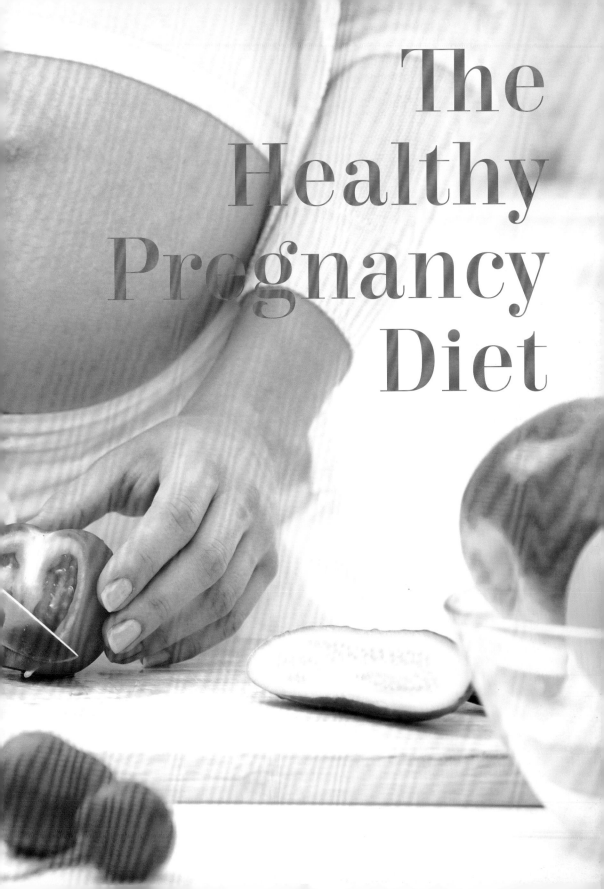

The
Healthy
Pregnancy
Diet

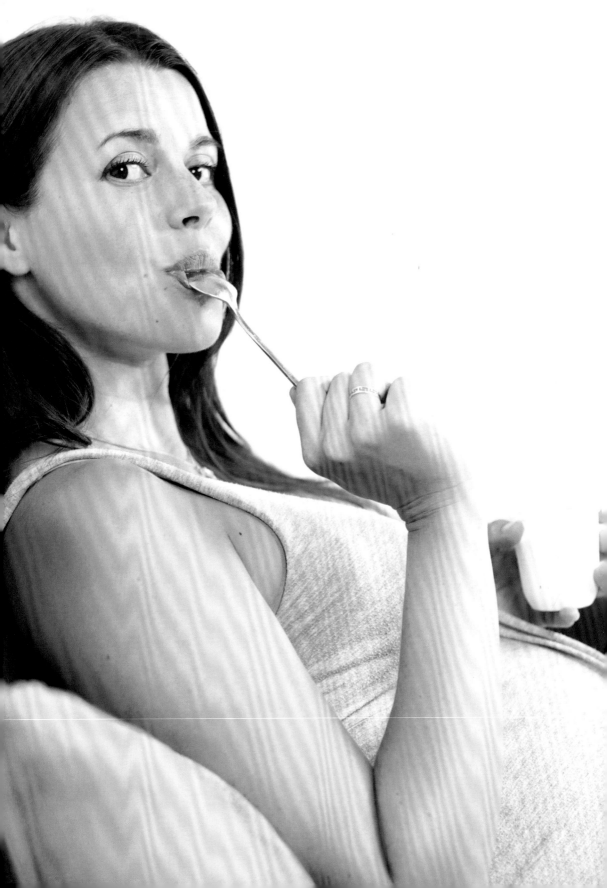

At no other time in your life is your diet more important than when you are pregnant.

Simply put, the diet you choose during pregnancy is not only highly influential to your own health and wellbeing, but also to the health, both present and future, of the completely dependent person growing inside you.

Eating a wholesome, well-balanced diet is vital for expectant mums to reduce the likelihood of developing a number of common pregnancy complaints such as constipation, anaemia and gestational diabetes. Eating well will also help prevent putting on excessive weight during pregnancy, and help keep energy levels buoyant. Thus, good nutrition will seriously improve your chances of a joyous and fulfilling pregnancy experience.

But it can be difficult to eat healthily all the time, especially in the early stages of pregnancy if you have morning sickness, and when certain cravings take hold. Don't think that you need to be a martyr to nutritional perfection during these tough times. Rather, you should take a pragmatic approach and simply 'broaden' your dietary habits while you attempt to minimise the impact of cravings and the turn-offs of morning sickness.

There is no better time than pregnancy to switch to a diet rich in wholesome, unprocessed foods. Foods in their natural state are free from excessively high levels of sugars, salt and fats, along with nasty artificial additives. Variety is the key! Having a variety of nutritious foods means that you will get a wide array of important vitamins, minerals and antioxidants, as well as protein, complex carbohydrates and good fats, all of which you need for a healthy pregnancy and, of course, your baby's optimal growth and development.

Further to the concept of eating for your own sake, a great and simple rule of thumb is to always remember that everything you eat, your baby does too.

This single reminder will constantly help you check your choices and help you favour, on balance, those foods that are beneficial for both you and your baby.

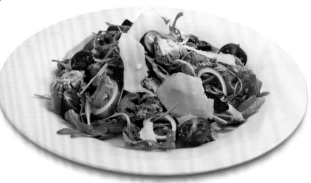

Simple Steps to a Healthier Pregnancy Diet

• Swap any 'white' refined grains (white breads, pasta, rice, crackers and products made with white flour) and processed sugary breakfast cereals for healthy, wholegrain varieties (grainy breads, wholemeal pasta and crackers, quinoa, brown rice, buckwheat, whole oats and muesli).

• Limit commercially made cakes, muffins and cookies and make your own healthy, high fibre, wholemeal versions.

• Include plenty of vegetables each day and have a good variety of different colours, don't forget your super brassica vegetables (broccoli, cauliflower, and cabbage). Vegetable juice is also an excellent way to increase your intake.

• Keep dried and tinned legumes in the house to make soups, hummus, dahl and salads.

• Eat a few pieces of fresh fruit each day. Add to fruit salads, smoothies, breakfast cereal, through yoghurt or as a snack. Small servings of dried fruit also make a healthy fibre-rich snack and are great mixed with raw nuts and seeds. Go easy on fruit juice though as it is high in fructose.

• Include low-fat dairy products such as yoghurt, cheese and milk in your diet. If you are lactose-intolerant, good alternatives are calcium-enriched rice and organic soy milk, almond milk, or lactose-free milk and yoghurt.

• Have a selection of raw nuts and seeds at home in a jar to snack on, or to add to breakfast cereals, smoothies and salads. Pure nut butters and tahini are also delicious spread on toast, sandwiches or crackers, or added to dips like hummus.

• Buy good quality organic chicken and eggs, lean meats and fish, and organic soy products (tofu, tempeh and miso).

• Buy healthy oils such as cold pressed virgin or extra virgin olive oil and coconut oil to cook with, and flaxseed, walnut and avocado oils to use over salads and breads.

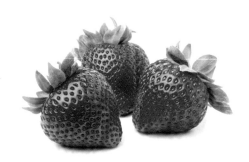

Top 10 Nutritional Tips for Expectant Mums

1 Totally abstain from drinking alcohol.

2 A majority of your diet should be made up of wholesome, unprocessed foods in their natural state; foods that are rich in nutrients and fibre. Limit any heavily processed or refined foods that are high in salt, sugars and bad fats.

3 Try to eat organic produce that is free from toxic pesticide and herbicide residue.

4 Take a good pregnancy multi-vitamin that contains 500mcg of folic acid daily.

5 Drink at least 2 litres of water daily.

6 Eat foods that contain essential omega-3 fats such as oily fish, nuts and seeds, and flaxseed oil, in addition to taking a good quality fish oil supplement.

7 Eat plenty of green, leafy vegetables that are rich in folic acid.

8 Include probiotic-rich foods in your daily diet such as yoghurt, and take a probiotic supplement (especially for your last trimester).

9 Eat smaller, healthier meals throughout the day, and make sure you include a couple of healthy protein-rich snacks.

10 Eat foods rich in iron including lean meat, fish, chicken, green leafy vegetables, seaweed and legumes.

7-*day* Healthy Pregnancy

	BREAKFAST	SNACK
MONDAY	Natural muesli with pumpkin and sunflower seeds, handful of mixed berries with milk	Tub of yoghurt with a piece of fruit
TUESDAY	Scrambled eggs with baby spinach and avocado on rye toast drizzled with flaxseed oil	Hummus with carrot and celery sticks and a piece of fruit
WEDNESDAY	Bircher muesli with almonds, grated apple, strawberry, chia seeds, and natural bio yoghurt	Handful of raw nuts and seeds and a vegetable juice (carrot, beetroot, celery, ginger, apple)
THURSDAY	Smoothie with milk, berries, frozen banana, LSA (ground linseeds, sunflower seeds, almonds), and natural bio yoghurt	Hummus with rice crackers and a piece of fruit
FRIDAY	Whole oat porridge with banana, cinnamon, flaked almonds, dollop of natural bio yoghurt and a drizzle of raw honey	Rice cakes with almond butter and sliced banana
SATURDAY	Omelette with fresh basil, cherry tomatoes with wholegrain toast drizzled with flaxseed oil	Banana protein smoothie with milk, yoghurt, chia seeds, and a little raw honey
SUNDAY	Natural muesli with almond milk, diced pear, strawberries, and linseeds	Hummus with crackers and a vegetable juice

Meal Planner

LUNCH	SNACK	DINNER
Beetroot and pumpkin salad with chickpeas, walnuts, baby spinach and lemon juice and flaxseed oil dressing	Puffed rice cakes with cottage cheese, avocado and tomato slices	Grilled salmon fillet with steamed broccoli and baby carrots, with baked sweet potato chips
Chicken and salad sandwich with wholegrain mustard on grainy bread	Handful of trail mix: raw nuts, seeds and sun-dried fruits	Beef stir-fry with ginger, broccoli, red capsicum and carrot with brown rice and sesame seeds
Lentil and green bean salad with cherry tomatoes, celery, pumpkin seeds, parsley and lemon juice. A piece of grainy toast with avocado	Cheese and tomato on wholegrain crackers with a piece of fruit	Vegetable frittata with mixed greens and avocado salad
Salmon salad with green leaves, cucumber, tomato, avocado and lemon juice	Yoghurt topped with nuts and blueberries	Organic tofu and vegetable curry with quinoa topped with sunflower seeds
Toasted hummus and roast vegetable wholemeal wrap with baby spinach	Handful of raw mixed nuts and seeds with a vegetable juice	Grilled organic chicken breast with steamed snow peas, carrots, baby corn, and baby potatoes
Diced roast vegetables and cous cous salad topped with Greek yoghurt	Wholemeal crackers with cottage cheese, avocado and tomato slices	Salmon fish cakes with steamed mixed greens and baby carrots
Sourdough sandwich with turkey, rocket, tomato and raw grated beetroot	Small tub of yoghurt with handful of raw nuts	Lamb cutlets with steamed vegetables and baked sweet potato wedges

Organic foods are the best in pregnancy

All mums-to-be want their babies to have the very best start in life, and one important way they can do this is by eating healthy, organic foods that are free from toxins such as pesticides and herbicides, growth hormones, genetically modified ingredients, and other chemical additives and preservatives. Pesticide and herbicide residue remains on commercially-grown crops, which ultimately end up on your dinner plate and could potentially affect your health and the health of your growing baby.

The consumption of commercially-grown foods produced using pesticides and hormones has been linked to a number of adverse health effects, especially in unborn babies who are most vulnerable to the effects of these types of toxins.

There is increasing evidence that prenatal exposure to pesticides may have health impacts on a child later in life. Researchers at the University of California have recently found that prenatal exposure to organophosphate pesticides, widely used on food crops, is related to lower intelligence scores in early childhood. [1]

Organic foods are not only better for you and your baby's health, they taste better and generally have higher levels of nutrients, especially antioxidants, compared to commercially grown crops.

Another bonus of buying organic fruits and vegetables is that you can eat their edible skins, which are an excellent source of dietary fibre. This is a great way to further boost your fibre intake to prevent pregnancy constipation.

It is also a good idea to buy organic red meat, chicken, eggs, and cow's milk. Organic livestock are fed organic feed and are not given antibiotics or hormones. Organic milk is also richer in beneficial omega-3 fats, which are essential for a growing baby's brain development.

Ideally, you should aim to buy organic as much as possible. Not everyone, however, can afford to go 100% organic all of the time, or has access to organic produce regularly. Unfortunately, organic foods can be a little more expensive, especially in supermarkets and health food stores. It's a good idea to check if you have an organic farmers market in your local neighbourhood. Not only will you be supporting your local small farmers but it's usually cheaper too.

For those times when you can't go 100% organic, you can prioritise your selection of organic foods to those that are most susceptible to higher levels of pesticide residues:

- Thin skinned berries, tomatoes, peaches, cherries and grapes.

- Green leafy vegetables.

- Soy products.

- Apples and cucumbers with wax coatings, carrots and potatoes.

- Red meat, chicken, eggs and cow's milk.

Tips for preparing non-organic produce

- Wash all non-organic fruits and vegetables well.

- Peel off skin.

- Rinse rice, grains and legumes well and use clean water to cook with.

- Trim any visible fat from meat.

- Lamb generally contains less toxins than other types of meat so is a good choice.

Grazing eat smaller meals more often

Grazing on smaller, healthy meals and snacks throughout the day is definitely the best approach when you are pregnant. Eating smaller meals will help reduce the risk of suffering from common pregnancy digestive problems such as indigestion and heartburn.

A lot of women with morning sickness say it really helps for them to snack throughout the day, as having something in their stomach alleviates the nausea.

Another good reason to be a grazer is that it will help keep your blood sugar levels balanced. If you go for too long without food, your blood sugar levels could drop, leaving you feeling tired and craving sugary foods in an attempt to bring your levels up. Grazing will provide you with a steady supply of glucose for energy and other important nutrients your baby needs for optimal growth and development.

You should be aiming to have a healthy breakfast, lunch and dinner with a couple of protein-rich snacks in between.

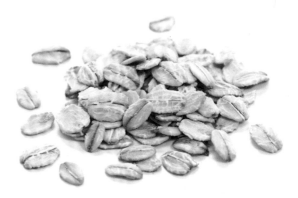

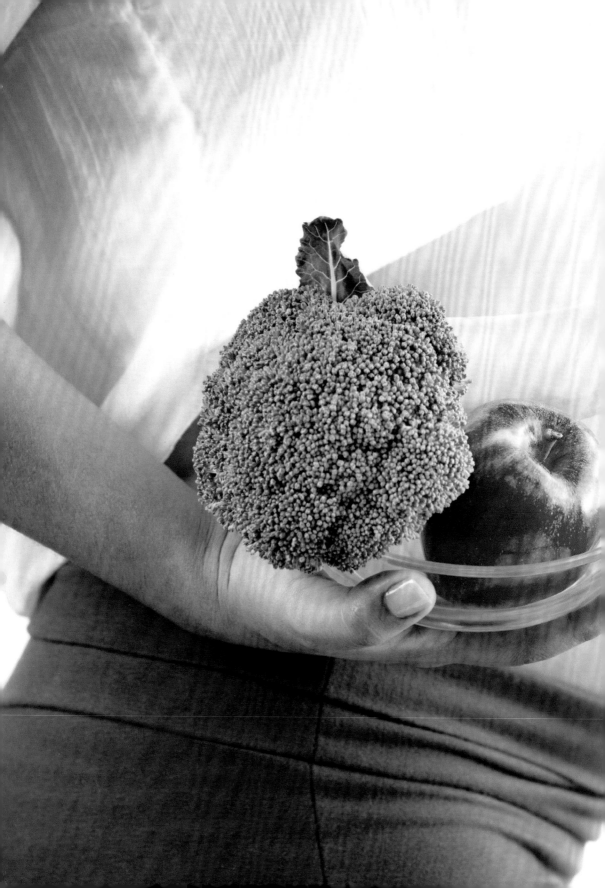

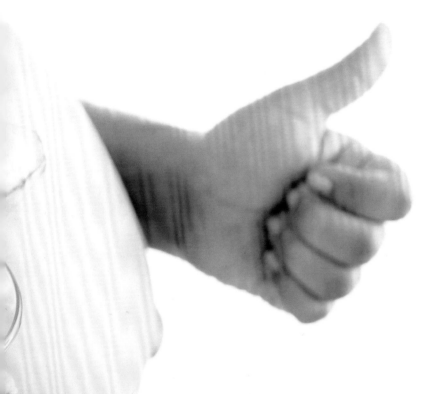

Pregnancy
Superfoods

Berries
bursting with antioxidants

Bright, beautiful berries are one of the best sources of protective antioxidants and are an excellent addition to any pregnant woman's diet. Their rich red, blue and purple colours indicate the presence of high levels of anthocyanins, which is a powerful antioxidant that helps protect from damaging free radicals. Antioxidants help protect us from chronic diseases such as cancers, heart disease, diabetes, and from premature aging.

Berries are also a brilliant source of vitamin C, which pregnant women need good levels of to help support immune function and decrease the risk of infections.

Your baby also needs plenty of vitamin C for collagen production and for optimal growth and development.

Including berries in your daily diet will help boost your fibre intake to prevent constipation in pregnancy. A handful of berries mixed through a small tub of yoghurt, or used in a smoothie, are two highly nutritious low GI snacks.

If you haven't tried acai berries yet they are definitely worth a try. These little purple berries from the Amazon certainly pack a punch when it comes to antioxidants. Acai berries have an impressive 42 times the antioxidant concentration of blueberries.

Super purple berries

If you haven't tried super purple berries from the Amazon yet you should definitely give them a go. Acai, Maqui and Camu Camu berries have exceptionally high levels of anthocynanins, which are highly effective antioxidants. These berries have much higher antioxidant levels than other well known antioxidant-rich foods like blueberries.

Pregnant women need plenty of antioxidants in their daily diet for protection against oxidative stress, cell damage and for improved immune function. These super berries are also a superb source of vitamin C, which is brilliant for fighting off infections, along with being essential for a baby's growth and development. Pregnant women are a lot more susceptible to coming down with colds, the flu and other infections due to pregnancy hormones suppressing their immune systems.

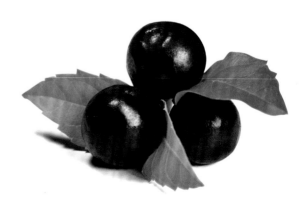

Coconut oil

This incredibly nourishing super food is a wonderful addition to the diet, especially during pregnancy. Coconut oil - made from the flesh of mature coconuts - contains nutrients and beneficial fatty acids that offer expectant mums and their babies many wonderful health benefits, including protection against infections. Fat is vital for a healthy pregnancy and breastfeeding experience, however it needs to be the right type of fat. Natural, unrefined saturated fats, such as those found in coconut oil, are a wonderful addition to a pregnant woman's diet. It is the refined hydrogenated trans fats found in processed and junk foods that should be avoided. We need saturated fats to produce cholesterol, necessary for the formation of healthy cell membranes, and to make hormones, essential for a healthy pregnancy.

Coconut oil is a rich source of lauric and capric acid: rare fatty acids also found in breast milk. These beneficial fatty acids have potent anti-microbial properties, which boost immunity and help to protect mother and baby from bacterial, viral and fungal infections. Coconut oil is particularly beneficial for preventing and treating candida, which is a common complaint in pregnancy.

Coconut oil is also ideal for breastfeeding mums. The healthy fats found in coconut milk are beneficial for improving milk production. Studies have also shown that mums who include coconut oil in their diet have much higher levels of protective lauric and capric acid in their breast milk.[2]

Coconut oil contains medium chain fatty acids (MCFA), which is a type of saturated fat that behaves differently from other fats. MCFA fats can be absorbed straight into the cell where it can immediately be burned up as energy, making it a fabulous energy source to support a baby's rapid growth. Adding coconut oil to the diet can also help balance blood sugar levels, which helps reduce the risk of gestational diabetes, along with supporting pregnant women's health by boosting energy levels and promoting a healthy weight.

Coconut oil is incredibly nourishing for the inside and out. Not only can you eat coconut oil when you're pregnant but it is also great to put on your skin.

It is extremely moisturising and can help to prevent stretch marks and reduce itching. It is also ideal for rubbing on nipples while breastfeeding to prevent cracking and soreness. Then once you've had your baby, coconut oil is an excellent choice for their delicate skin, preventing and treating nappy rash and cradle cap and for relaxing baby massages.

The best way to include coconut oil in your diet is to add 1 tablespoon to smoothies or porridges. Use it in place of vegetable oils or butter to cook with, or to use in baked goods. Coconut oil has a higher tolerance to heat compared to other oils so it won't turn into harmful trans fat, making it a healthy choice for stir frying and baking. You can make delicious raw snacks and desserts using coconut oil, which are included in this book.

Fresh vegetable juices

Fresh vegetable juices are packed with nourishing vitamins, minerals, living enzymes and antioxidants, which are essential for a healthy pregnancy and baby.

Juices are easy for the body to digest and absorb, so you can deliver high levels of vitamins and minerals to you and your baby's cells. Juicing is also an excellent way to increase your vegetable intake.

By juicing a variety of different coloured vegetables you will ensure that you are getting a nice array of important pregnancy nutrients. Blue, purple and red produce are rich in antioxidants, orange varieties are high in beta-carotene, and green, leafy vegetables are rich in iron, vitamin K, folate and calcium. Add a little fruit to your juices for taste and for an extra boost in antioxidants and immune boosting vitamin C.

Always choose organic fruits and vegetables when you can, so that your juice will be free from pesticides but bursting with flavour and nutritional goodness. Vegetables that juice well are carrots (orange and purple), beetroot, celery, cucumber, broccoli, spinach, baby spinach, kale, lettuce and herbs like parsley, mint and coriander. If you are new to juicing vegetables add around 30-40% fruit to start. Fruits that combine well with vegetables include apples, pears, lemon, grapefruit, kiwi fruit and berries. Experiment with different combinations. Drinking too much fruit juice can affect blood sugar levels, due to their high fructose concentration. Although fructose is naturally occurring, when fibre has been removed, such as in juice, fructose acts like sugar in the body causing havoc with blood sugar levels. A little fresh fruit juice added to a veggie juice is healthy; drinking just fruit juice regularly is not.

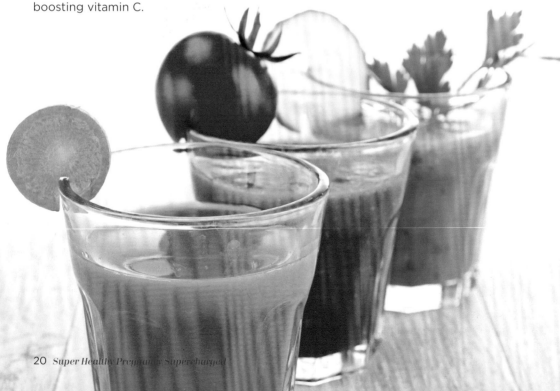

Organic eggs
packed full of goodness

Scrambled, boiled, or made into a frittata or quiche, eggs are extremely versatile and full of nutritional goodness. They are rich in protein and provide plenty of amino acids to support the growth of your baby. Eggs are also a good source of vitamin B12, which is important for your baby's nervous system and brain development, as well as supporting your need to make extra red blood cells.

Eggs have been found to be one of the few foods that are a naturally good source of vitamin D.

They provide around 41iu of vitamin D per large yolk, essential for your baby's healthy bone formation.

Eggs also contain choline (also found in the yolk) that is important for foetal and infant brain development, and is needed to make the neurotransmitter acetylcholine, which is vital for nervous system function.

The old concern about eggs and cholesterol levels is somewhat overstated. In fact, you need not worry about your cholesterol levels with a moderate consumption of eggs in the diet. Researchers have found that you can enjoy eating an egg a day without any concern of raising your cholesterol levels.

Pregnant women should choose organic eggs when possible and make sure that the eggs are cooked well. Undercooked eggs could possibly contain salmonella, which has been linked to miscarriage or other pregnancy complications.

Fermented brown rice protein powders

Pregnant women need an increased supply of protein throughout their pregnancy to support their baby's rapid growth, as well as their own increase in blood volume. Fermented brown rice protein powders are a lovely way to easily add more plant-based protein to the diet. They are an excellent source of high quality protein, containing around 80% pure protein. The fermenting process also increases the levels of essential and non-essential amino acids, and also boosts B vitamins and other important pregnancy minerals such as iron, calcium, and magnesium. Brown rice protein powders are also a great source of fibre, to help promote good bowel health and prevent constipation. Including this form of protein into the diet is a great way to help stabalise blood sugar levels and also curb sugar cravings, which can help reduce the risk of mothers developing gestational diabetes. It is also easily digested and great for anyone who is sensitive to dairy. Brown rice protein powder is extremely versatile, and can be added easily to smoothies, breakfast cereals, and protein balls and bars.

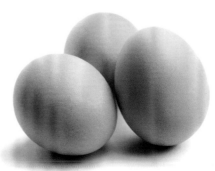

Seaweed
super sea vegetable

Another superfood that can really help boost health and nutritional intake is seaweed. Seaweed is abundant in many nutrients women need for a healthy pregnancy and baby. Being a great source of zinc and antioxidants, seaweed helps support immune function and has anti-cancerous properties. It can help boost energy levels and support red blood cell production due to its vitamin B and iron content.

Seaweed is your best source of iodine, which is particularly important for supporting your baby's developing brain and nervous system.

This superfood is also beneficial for managing healthy blood sugar levels, and is a good source of protein, chromium and magnesium, which can reduce the risk of gestational diabetes. Seaweed will also help promote healthy blood clotting as it's packed with vitamin K.

There are many different types of seaweed to choose from including kelp, nori, and akrame. It is delicious added to soups, salads and stir-fries.

Garlic
enhance your immunity

Expectant mums are more vulnerable to colds, flu and infections, such as urinary tract infections and thrush, as their immune function is weakened during pregnancy.

One of the best ways to strengthen your immune system naturally is to include garlic in the diet. Garlic is a safe and effective way to prevent or treat colds and flu and other infections during pregnancy as it has strong anti-bacterial, fungal and viral action. Garlic contains sulphur compounds that have potent immune-enhancing and antioxidant actions. Garlic is also a good source of vitamins A, C, selenium, and zinc, which all play pivotal roles in immune function. Another benefit of eating garlic while pregnant is that it can help lower blood pressure.

Overcooking can destroy a lot of garlic's antioxidant properties so you are best to eat garlic raw in dips like hummus, or add garlic in cooking closer to the end. Garlic tablets can be very helpful for treating colds and flu.

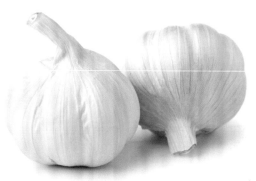

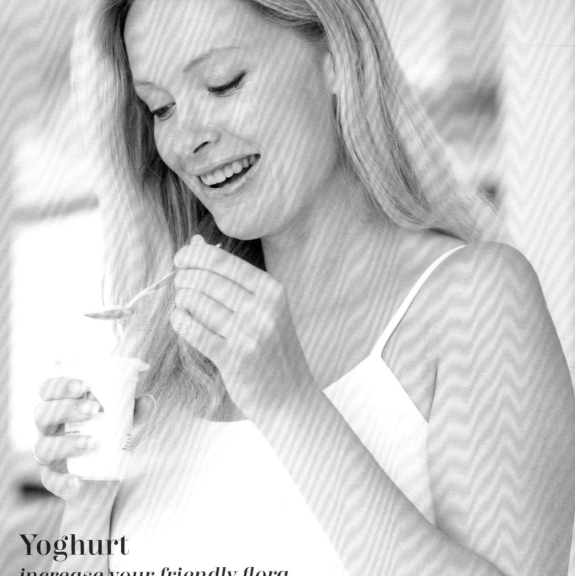

Yoghurt
increase your friendly flora

Yoghurt is the perfect protein-rich snack, ideal for helping keep blood sugar levels balanced and sugar cravings at bay. Yoghurt will supply you with plenty of calcium and vitamin D, which your baby needs for optimal bone growth, and B vitamins (including B12), which is important for red blood cell production and your baby's nervous system development.

Yoghurt also has the ability to promote healthy immune function and digestion due to the presence of beneficial bacteria, which help promote a healthy balance of bowel flora.

When buying yoghurt make sure it has 'live or active bacteria' on the label, and watch out for yoghurts with lots of added sugars. Some yoghurt can contain 4 - 5 teaspoons of added sugar per small tub.

Ginger
more than a morning sickness cure

Ginger is most widely-know for its ability to relieve nausea and vomiting associated with morning sickness. A lot of women find sipping on ginger tea, or taking ginger tablets can help ease their nausea. Ginger is also useful for relieving indigestion and improving circulation, which can become sluggish during pregnancy.

Ginger is rich in antioxidants and helps support healthy immune function. It's also a safe and natural alternative to use if you have a cold during pregnancy, as it helps relieve congestion and sore throats.

Ginger can be easily added to vegetable juices, or thrown into stir-fries and curries.

Morning sickness

When you talk to pregnant women, the term 'morning sickness' is quickly waved-off as a rather lame description of what many of them have to endure. Try expressions like 'all-day-and-all-night sickness' or 'never ending sea-sickness' and you start to get a picture of what it is really like for many. Most get by on willpower, fuelled by the notion that morning sickness doesn't last forever and that the wonderful endpoint of a bouncing bundle of joy clearly outweighs any illness along the way.

Around two thirds of all pregnant women tend to suffer from morning sickness, particularly in the first trimester. It generally starts around week 4 - 6 and usually lasts until week 12 - 14. As the name suggests, morning sickness is generally worse in the morning, although a lot of women feel sick all through the day. Then there are some women who suffer from severe morning sickness (hyperemesis gravidarum) throughout their entire pregnancy. This only affects a minority but does require close medical supervision.

Food can be the last thing on your mind when you are feeling nauseous. On some days it can be difficult to stomach anything. You not only lose your appetite, you sometimes can't even stand the sight or smell of foods you once loved. And then some women start craving weird and wonderful things they would never normally eat. It can be common for mums to lose weight in the first few months of pregnancy due to this.

Have faith though. These abnormal appetites and attitudes to food and the nausea itself usually pass at the end of the first trimester, and then most mums start feeling fantastic and get that much anticipated pregnancy glow. Ultimately, they also put any weight they may have lost back on again.

There are a few different factors that can contribute to morning sickness including increased pregnancy hormone levels (mainly oestrogen), low blood sugar levels and changes in smell and taste.

There is an upside. There are potent natural means to help relieve your symptoms of morning sickness. Of course, different things work for different mums. Some of these tips work wonderfully for some and are less effective for others so make sure to give all of them a go if your morning sickness is proving difficult to manage.

- Nausea is aggravated by hypoglycaemia (low blood sugar levels). Often eating something light helps ease the nausea. Having snacks on hand throughout the day is one way to help keep blood sugar levels stable. Nibbling on dry crackers or toast when feeling queasy or keeping something by the bed if you wake up feeling nauseous through the night is a good idea. Some good protein choices include a small tub of yoghurt, a handful of trail mix (nuts and seeds), hummus, cheese or almond butter on a cracker or piece of toast.

- Avoid having an empty stomach as this usually makes women feel worse. Eating smaller meals more frequently will also help keep blood sugar levels more stable.

- Ginger works well for alleviating morning sickness too. Add a few slices of fresh ginger in a cup of boiling water or use a ginger tea bag; let it infuse for 10 minutes, then drink. Or, try making up a large jug of homemade ginger tea and drink it throughout the day cold. Ginger tablets are another good option to ease morning sickness, however do not exceed 2000 mg/day. Some women find relief from chewing on crystallised ginger.

- Taking a magnesium and vitamin B6 nutritional supplement can help reduce nausea and vomiting associated with pregnancy.

- It is important that you stay well hydrated, especially if you are unlucky enough to be vomiting. Having too much water in one go can make some women feel sick so just take sips of water regularly throughout the day. Women who are unable to keep any food or water down and are vomiting excessively should contact their doctor, to make sure they are not at risk of dehydration or nutritional deficiencies.

- Pregnant women have a heightened sense of smell and may be sensitive to certain odours, which make them feel nauseous. Avoiding certain strong smelling odours such as garlic, onions, and perfumes can be key to minimising nausea. Some women find it useful to have a nice smelling, soothing cream in their bag to put on and smell to help alleviate nausea from other smells.

- Make your own healthy icy poles with fruit juice and water and suck on them throughout the day.

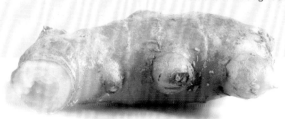

Spirulina
super algae

This superfood is an excellent source of easily digested, high quality protein to supply your baby with the essential amino acids they need for optimal growth and development. Being a good source of protein and magnesium, spirulina helps stabilise blood sugar levels and curb sugar cravings, making it ideal for reducing the risk of gestational diabetes. Spirulina is also a good source of beta-carotene for your baby's healthy eye development and immune function, and B12 for its nervous system development.

This health-promoting algae is one of the best sources of gamma-linolenic acid (GLA), an omega-3 essential fatty acid necessary for healthy brain and heart function. GLA is also found abundantly in mother's milk.

Spirulina is particularly beneficial for pregnant women who have low iron levels, being a very good source of easily absorbable iron, and B vitamins including folate, to help prevent neural tube defects and give pregnant women a much needed boost in energy. Spirulina is also useful for increasing vitamin K levels in pregnant women to promote healthy blood clotting.

A good maintenance dose during pregnancy is 5 - 6 capsules daily or 1 heaped teaspoon of powder in a fresh fruit and vegetable juice, smoothie or water. Spirulina has a seaweed-like smell so if you are already feeling a little queasy then capsules are probably a better option.

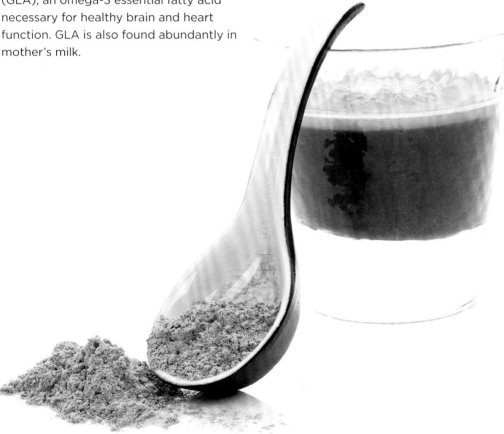

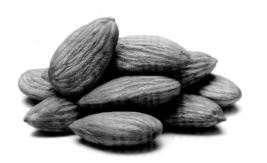

Almonds
the perfect protein snack

A handful of almonds is the perfect way to satisfy those afternoon munchies. Packed with protein and other important pregnancy nutrients, these nuts sure do pack a nutritional punch. Almonds are a great source of calcium for your baby's bone development, with 28g containing as much calcium as a quarter of a cup of milk. Almonds also contain zinc to help support you and your baby's immune function, and vitamin E, which is a potent antioxidant. Almonds are also a good source of heart healthy monounsaturated fats, and folic acid, which is essential during pregnancy to prevent neural tube defects.

Pumpkin and sunflower seeds
versatile and highly nutritious

A great healthy snack for mums-to-be, perfect mixed with nuts and sun-dried fruit, or added to breakfast cereals or salads. These seeds will provide you with plenty of nutrients needed for a healthy pregnancy and baby, namely zinc, which will help prevent stretch marks and support healthy immune function and wound healing after birth.

Being rich in protein, these seeds will provide your baby with the essential amino acids they need for optimal growth and development, as well as helping keep blood sugar levels balanced and sugar cravings at bay. These seeds also contain vitamin E and selenium, which are both potent antioxidants, iron needed for red blood cell production, and magnesium to help boost mum's energy levels.

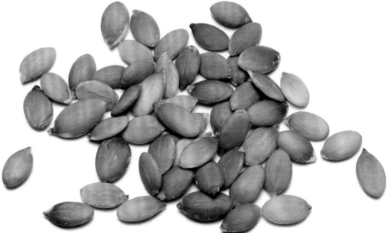

Salmon
baby brain food

Pregnant mums-to-be and their babies will benefit greatly from including salmon 2 - 3 times a week in their diet. Salmon, like other oily fish, contains high levels of beneficial omega-3 essential fatty acids and DHA (docosahexaenoic acid), which is the main component of brain cell membranes.

These healthy fats are vital for baby's normal brain and eye development during pregnancy and while breastfeeding.

Eating fish during pregnancy has been shown to improve your child's intelligence. According to a recent study published in the American Journal of Clinical Nutrition infants of mothers who consumed more fish during pregnancy received higher scores in verbal intelligence and fine motor skill tests and had better pro-social behaviour. [3]

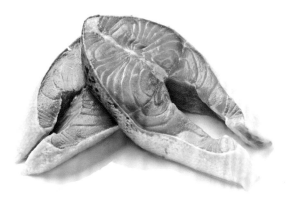

Salmon is an excellent choice of fish for pregnant women as it contains low levels of heavy metals such as mercury, and high levels of omega-3 fats. Salmon is rich in protein to supply plenty of amino acids to support your baby's growth and development and your increasing red blood cell production. Salmon will also provide you with plenty of zinc, which is an important mineral for your baby's bone and brain formation, together with giving both mum and baby's immune system a boost.

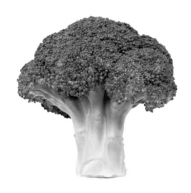

Broccoli
brilliant brassicas

Broccoli is an excellent source of vitamin C, which your baby needs for collagen production. It provides you with lots of beta-carotene for baby's eye development and healthy eyesight, along with good doses of folic acid, which decreases the chances of your baby being born with spina bifida. Eating broccoli regularly will help boost your fibre intake, as well as improve your liver's ability to detoxify and reduce the risk of cancers and other chronic diseases.

Green leafy vegetables
boost your folate

Green leafy vegetables are an excellent source of the B vitamin folate, which can decrease the risk of neural tube defects such as spina bifida. Rich in important vitamins, minerals and health promoting antioxidants, these nutritional powerhouses are one of the most nutrient dense foods around.

They're also rich in calcium, which your baby needs to build strong, healthy bones and teeth. A cup of dandelion greens contains more calcium than half a cup of milk. There are some varieties however, such as Swiss chard, collards, spinach and beet greens that should not be relied on for their calcium content as they contain high levels of oxalates, compounds that block calcium absorption.

Many green leafy vegetables, especially spinach and Swiss chard, are good sources of iron, which pregnant women need be able to produce the extra blood needed to nourish a growing baby.

Green leafy vegetables are also an excellent source of vitamin K, which helps regulate blood clotting.

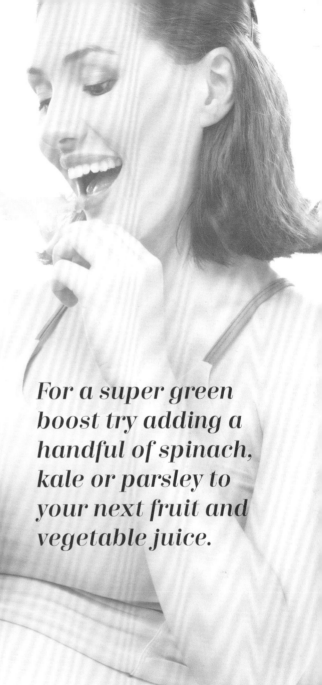

For a super green boost try adding a handful of spinach, kale or parsley to your next fruit and vegetable juice.

Avocado
good fats for good health

Avocado's smooth, buttery flesh is an excellent source of heart-healthy fats and vitamin E, which is essential for supporting your baby's nervous system, as well as beta-carotene for eye development and good vision.

Avocados also contain B vitamins such as folate, which are necessary to help prevent neural tube defects, and more potassium than a medium banana, to keep mum's blood pressure at a healthy level. Make sure you also eat the darker green flesh that is closest to the skin as it contains the most nutrients.

Tahini
step up your calcium intake

Tahini is a highly nutritious paste made from ground sesame seeds that contains plenty of calcium to support the growth of your baby's bones and teeth. Tahini also provides plenty of healthy unsaturated fats and vitamin E. Unhulled tahini, made with whole sesame seeds, is richer in calcium and other nutrients compared to the hulled variety, although it does have a slightly bitter taste. Expectant mums will benefit from including tahini in their diet, as it's a rich source of protein and amino acids. Tahini is very versatile, delicious spread on toast or on sandwiches, added to dips like hummus or in salad dressings.

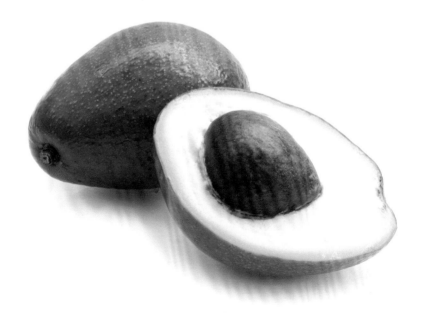

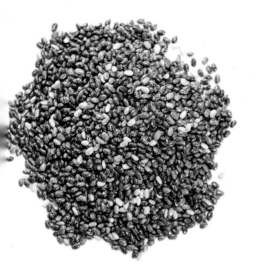

Chia seeds
super healthy

They may be tiny but they're big on nutritional value. Chia seeds are the richest plant source of alpha-linolenic acid, a type of omega-3 fat, which the body uses to make DHA. These beneficial fats are vital for supporting your baby's brain development and function, as well as helping keep women's skin soft and supple and less likely to develop stretch marks. Chia seeds are an excellent source of fibre to help keep expectant mums free from constipation, and provide protein and calcium to help support your baby's healthy bone development. Try adding a spoonful of chia seeds to your breakfast cereal, smoothie or yoghurt.

Quinoa
the mother grain

Quinoa (pronounced keen-wa) is technically a seed grown from a grain-like crop, however it is commonly considered a wholegrain as it can be used just like other grains. Quinoa is one of the most nutritious grains around, containing more protein than any other grain. This gluten-free grain is a great source of iron, helping support a pregnant woman's need for extra red blood cells and prevent anaemia. Half a cup of quinoa contains 4mg of iron. This nutritious grain also provides good levels of calcium, B vitamins, and vitamin E.

Expectant mums need to eat plenty of fibre-rich foods such as quinoa to keep them regular and constipation free. Quinoa also has a low GI so it's a perfect grain for keeping blood sugar levels stable and for reducing the risk of gestational diabetes.

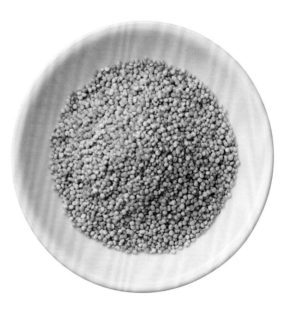

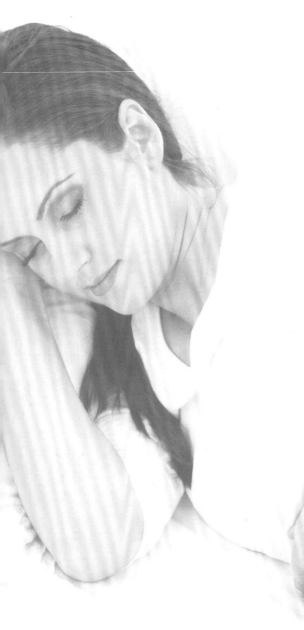

Whole oats
energy to fuel your day

One of the best ways you can start the day is with a nourishing bowl of porridge or muesli. Oats are a superb source of slow releasing complex carbohydrates, which supply you with sustained energy throughout the day. Oats are also abundant in a host of important nutrients women need for a healthy pregnancy and baby.

Oats are rich in magnesium, which can help alleviate pregnancy complaints such as leg cramps, morning sickness, and fluid retention. Your baby also needs plenty of magnesium for their bone, teeth and nervous system development. Oats are also a good source of the powerful antioxidant selenium, which will help support you and your baby's immune function.

Oats are used by herbalists to calm, support and nourish the nervous system, which is ideal for expectant mums who are feeling tired, stressed and having trouble sleeping.

Choose whole oats over the quick cook variety as they are richer in fibre and nutritional goodness. Whole oats are a fantastic source of both insoluble, to help keep you regular, and the soluble fibre beta-glucan, which helps protect you from cardiovascular disease and also helps keep blood sugar levels stable, reducing the risk of gestational diabetes. Beta-glucan is also thought to enhance immune function.

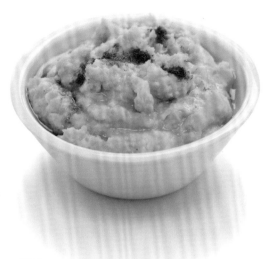

Hummus
nutritious snack staple

This tasty dip would have to be one of the healthiest protein-rich snacks around. Eaten with vegetable sticks, or on wholegrain crackers or toast, hummus provides plenty of protein to help support the growth of your baby, and fibre to help keep pregnant mums regular.

Hummus is a great source of iron, zinc, calcium, B vitamins, and beneficial unsaturated fats, which are all essential nutrients needed for a healthy baby and pregnancy.

Lentils
nutritional powerhouses

Lentils are one of the richest sources of folate, which you need in good amounts during pregnancy to reduce the risk of neural tube defects. Half a cup of cooked lentils provides 180mcg of folate, which is nearly half the daily recommended dosage.

Lentils are also an excellent source of protein. Pregnant women need extra protein to supply their baby with all the amino acids it needs for optimal growth. Lentils are also a fantastic source of dietary fibre, to help keep expectant mums free from constipation and haemorrhoids. Eating protein-rich lentils will also help keep your blood sugar levels balanced and sugar cravings at bay.

Lentils are delicious mixed through salads, rice dishes, dahls, vegetable patties and soups.

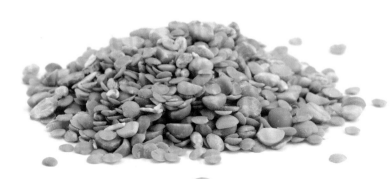

Beetroot
get juicing

Beetroot's vibrant purple pigment contains powerful antioxidants that help protect baby and mum from free radical damage, as well as reducing the risk of cancers and other chronic diseases.

This highly nutritious root vegetable is packed with beta-carotene and vitamin C, which pregnant mums need to give their immune systems a much needed boost, as well as folate and iron, required for red blood cell production and to reduce the risk of anaemia.

Fresh, raw beetroot is best grated into salads, on sandwiches and is delicious added to vegetable juices.

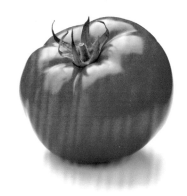

Tomatoes
antioxidant goodness

Red tomatoes are known for being the richest source of lycopene around, which acts as a very powerful antioxidant to protect mother and baby from damaging effects of free radicals, and to help ward off diseases such as heart disease and cancers.

Tomatoes also contain plenty of vitamin C and beta-carotene to strengthen a woman's immune function during pregnancy and protect them and their baby from infections. Tomatoes also provide you with good levels of potassium to help keep your blood pressure in check and help prevent leg cramps.

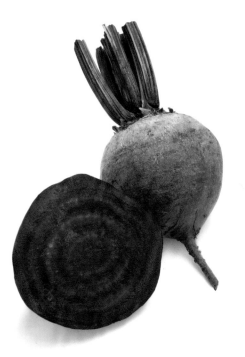

Do I need to eat for two? How much should I be eating?

Many women are under the misconception that as soon as they fall pregnant they have the green light to start eating for two. As tempting as this sounds, expectant mums don't need to double their food intake. It is actually your nutrient intake that needs to double during pregnancy not your calorie intake. So it is important for pregnant mums to eat wholesome foods that are nutrient-rich, along with the appropriate nutritional supplementation.

It's during the second trimester when women should increase their food intake by around 20%, and this should be made up by good quality, protein-rich foods. You could do this by including a couple of healthy protein-rich snacks during the day, such as a handful of raw nuts and seeds, hummus with wholegrain crackers or vegetable sticks, a small tub of yoghurt, a boiled egg, almond butter on toast, or a fruit protein smoothie. Your baby needs a constant supply of protein to support its rapidly growing body. Proteins are the building blocks for your baby's muscles, organs, skin and all other tissues in their body.

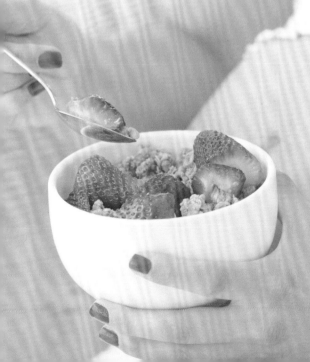

How much weight should I be putting on?

You shouldn't get too hung up on how much weight you've gained during pregnancy, as long as you are eating healthy foods and getting regular exercise (within your limits). It is a natural part of pregnancy to put on weight, and every woman is different, some putting on more than others. You do however want to try to stay within a healthy weight gain range, which can vary between 8 - 20kg (18 - 44 pounds). Although the average weight gain for expectant mums seems to be around 12 - 14kg (27 - 31 pounds). Most of your weight gain during pregnancy comes from the weight of your baby, placenta, amniotic fluid, breasts, and the increase in blood volume and fluid retention.

Women who are underweight before they fall pregnant can afford to put on extra weight, while women who were overweight before pregnancy should try not to put on more weight than the average. If you were carrying some extra weight before you fell pregnant, now is definitely not the time to go on a strict diet or to go hungry. Inadequate food intake may deprive your baby of important nutrients they need for optimal growth and development, and nutrients you need for a healthy pregnancy.

Gaining too much weight during pregnancy can lead to problems such as high blood pressure and problems with blood sugar levels, which can result in gestational diabetes. Pregnant women who are overweight also have an increased risk of having larger babies who put on weight more easily, and who have an increased risk of becoming overweight later in life.

Getting back into shape after your baby is born is often the last thing on your mind for a lot of mums, especially when they're sleep deprived, feeding around the clock, and learning the ropes of being a new mum. Maintaining a healthy weight during pregnancy will make it much easier to get back to your pre-baby shape.

If you are concerned that you are putting on too much weight talk to your nutritionist or naturopath, or get your midwife or doctor to put you in touch with a dietician at the hospital.

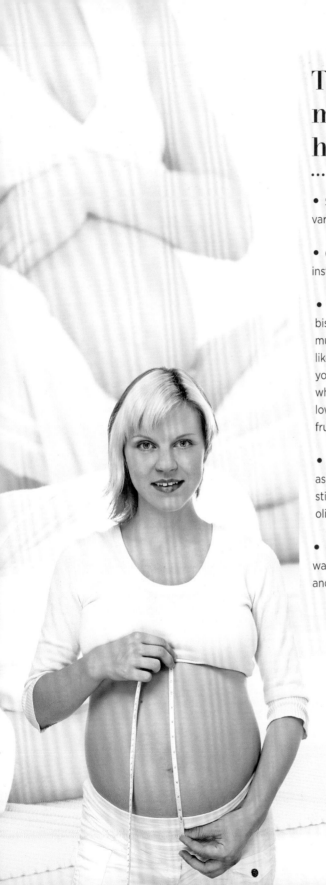

Tips for maintaining a healthy weight

••

• Swap full-fat dairy products for low-fat varieties.

• Opt for healthy homemade meals instead of greasy take-away.

• Cut down on sugary snacks such as biscuits, muffins, cake, confectionery and muesli bars. Choose protein-rich snacks like nuts, seeds and sun-dried fruits, yoghurt and fresh fruit, hummus and wholegrain crackers or vegetable sticks, low-fat cottage cheese on rice cakes, and fruit smoothies.

• Use healthy cooking techniques such as steaming, grilling and baking, and light stir-frying with healthy cooking oils like olive oil.

• Cut out soft drinks and go for water, sparkling mineral water, herbal teas and fresh vegetable and fruit juices.

Things to avoid during pregnancy

We are constantly being exposed to environmental toxins in our water supply, the air we breathe, and in the foods we eat, which can affect your health and the health of your unborn baby. There is no better time than now to give unhealthy habits the flick.

Eat safely

Food safety should be a concern for all expectant mums. Due to pregnancy hormones suppressing a woman's immune system, pregnant women are more vulnerable to food poisoning from food-borne infections such as salmonella, listeria and toxoplasma. Being infected will increase the risk of pregnancy complications such as miscarriage, stillbirth and premature labour.

What cheeses are safe for pregnant women?

Cheese is an important source of calcium for expectant mums, but certain kinds need to be avoided due to their higher risk of listeria infection. Cheeses made from pasteurised milk are fine; however cheeses made from raw unpasteurised milks are not safe to eat.

Soft cheeses are most likely to be made from unpasteurised milk, which includes feta, ricotta, brie, blue-veined cheese and camembert. These cheeses should be safe to eat, however, if well cooked.

All hard cheeses and the following soft and processed cheeses are safe to eat during pregnancy; cottage cheese, cream cheese, goat's cheese without white rind, mascarpone, Philadelphia, Quark and cheese spreads.

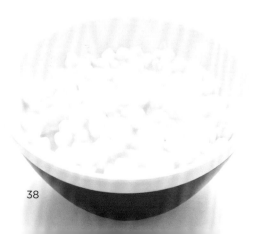

Listeria is a bacterium that can be very dangerous for pregnant women. Foods that can harbour listeria include unpasteurised and raw milk, soft cheeses, raw and undercooked or smoked seafood, deli meats, take away chicken salad and sandwiches, pre-prepared salads, and ready to eat processed foods that have not been heated to proper temperatures. Listeria is destroyed by the cooking process.

Toxoplasmosis can occur most commonly through touching cat faeces, when cleaning out cat litter or from contaminated soil in the garden. It could also occur from eating undercooked meats, or unwashed fruit and vegetables (especially from gardens with cats). Toxoplasmosis in pregnancy can lead to brain damage or blindness in your unborn baby. If you have a cat it is best to get someone else to clean the cat litter.

Salmonella infection can occur from eating raw unpasteurised milk, raw or undercooked meat, poultry or eggs, raw sprouts, salads (including chicken, tuna, potato), and cream desserts and fillings. Salmonella bacteria is destroyed by heating foods to 165°F or 74°C, and it can't grow at refrigerator or freezer temperatures.

Make some lifestyle changes and give your unhealthy habits the flick.

Reduce the risk of infection by following some simple food safety procedures

• Wash your hands well with soap and warm water after handling food, animals and after using the bathroom.

• Kitchen surfaces, cutting boards and utensils should be washed well before and after food preparation (especially after contact with raw meat, fish or poultry).

• Avoid eating raw or undercooked meat, poultry, fish or eggs.

• Reheat leftovers to 165°F or 74°C, and store all perishable foods below 40°F or 4°C. Freeze food if it's not going to be eaten within 4 days.

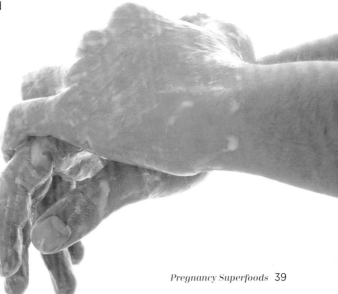

Alcohol

Latest guidelines and research suggest that there is NO safe level of alcohol consumption during pregnancy. The world health organization (WHO) and the national health and medical research council (NHMRC) both recommend that the only safe option is to completely abstain from drinking during pregnancy.

Alcohol is a toxin that can quickly travel from your bloodstream across the placenta barrier to your baby. Drinking alcohol regularly during pregnancy could not only cause miscarriage and premature birth, but can cause permanent damage to your developing baby.

Foetal alcohol syndrome is an irreversible and untreatable condition where babies develop unusual facial features, growth and development delays, poor coordination and learning difficulties, and behavioural problems, as a result of their mother drinking alcohol throughout pregnancy.

Damage to your baby from alcohol consumption can happen not just in the first trimester, as some women think, it can happen later when your baby's brain and nervous system is developing.

Alcohol also interferes with the absorption of certain important nutrients that are vital for your baby's health and for a healthy pregnancy, such as folic acid, vitamins A, D, E, C and K.

Illicit drugs

It may seem obvious but it is certainly worth emphasising that many illicit drugs such as marijuana (cannabis), cocaine, speed (amphetamines), crystal meth (methamphetamine), ecstasy, and heroin are considered very unsafe when consumed during pregnancy and will adversely affect both your health and the health of your unborn baby. These drugs pass through the placenta and can reduce the amount of oxygen and nutrients your baby receives, which will affect their growth and development.

Taking these drugs can also cause serious pregnancy complications such as placental abruption, where the placenta comes away from the uterus wall and can cause severe bleeding.

Perhaps most upsetting, babies born to mothers who have taken drugs regularly throughout their pregnancy may exhibit the often horrific symptoms of 'withdrawal' after birth.

Other effects of taking illicit drugs during pregnancy include giving birth to a low-birth weight baby, miscarriage, premature labour, increased risk of your baby being stillborn, or being born with heart problems. Some drugs can affect your baby's brain development and increase its risk of learning and behavioural problems in childhood.

Another danger of smoking during pregnancy is the increased risk of pregnancy complications such as miscarriage, placental abruption, premature labour and high blood pressure

Smoking

Every cigarette you smoke while you are pregnant will restrict the blood vessels to your baby, which will reduce the amount of oxygen and nutrients they receive. Not to mention the cocktail of dangerous chemicals that cross the placental barrier and are delivered straight to your unborn baby. Smoking will have a detrimental effect on your baby's growth and will greatly increase the risk of them being born a low-birth weight, and having respiratory problems such as asthma later on in life. Smoking also increases the risk of SIDS (Sudden infant death syndrome).

Another danger of smoking during pregnancy is the increased risk of pregnancy complications such as miscarriage, placental abruption, premature labour and high blood pressure. Smoking during breastfeeding is also dangerous as these harmful chemicals pass into your breast milk and can affect milk production.

Smoking can be extremely difficult for some people to give up, so if you are having trouble talk to your doctor or midwife. They will be able to provide you with numbers and information regarding quitting. Even passive smoking can affect your baby so make sure people don't smoke around you. Ideally both parents should stop smoking during pregnancy.

Pharmaceutical and herbal medications

Although some herbal medicines can be used safely during pregnancy, there are many herbs that are contraindicated in pregnancy, just like conventional medications. Some herbs could potentially be dangerous for your baby and may trigger premature contractions, so for this reason you should never self prescribe. Only take herbal medicines that have been prescribed by a qualified herbalist or naturopath, and to be on the safe side avoid all herbal medicines in the first trimester. Moderate amounts of culinary herbs and herbal teas, however, are considered safe in pregnancy.

While some conventional medications are considered safe during pregnancy, many aren't, or their effects are unknown. Before taking any medications ask your doctor.

Only take herbal medicines that have been prescribed by a qualified herbalist or naturopath

Caffeine

Do you rely on your morning coffee hit to kick start your day?

Maybe you should think again before you tuck into your next cup of coffee. Consuming too much caffeine in pregnancy is not recommended as it could negatively impact you and your growing baby's health.

Caffeine stimulates the production of the stress hormone cortisol, which can give you a much needed energy boost but can also make you feel anxious and edgy, and cause sleeping problems. Too much caffeine can also overstimulate your baby's nervous system. More than 300mg of caffeine a day, which is equivalent to drinking 3 coffees and a black tea, has been linked with miscarriage.

High levels of caffeine can increase your heart rate and blood pressure and can affect your blood sugar levels. Consuming too much caffeine may also affect you and your baby's bone health as it can decrease calcium absorption. It can also inhibit the absorption of iron, which is another important mineral during pregnancy.

Too much caffeine while breastfeeding is also not a good idea as it passes through your breast milk to your baby, which can make them over stimulated, irritable and more difficult to get to sleep.

The most common sources of caffeine are:

....

coffee (150-80mg per cup)

black tea (50mg per cup)

soft drink (40mg per can)

chocolate (20mg per 30g bar)

More than 300mg of caffeine a day, which is equivalent to drinking 3 coffees and a black tea, has been linked with miscarriage.

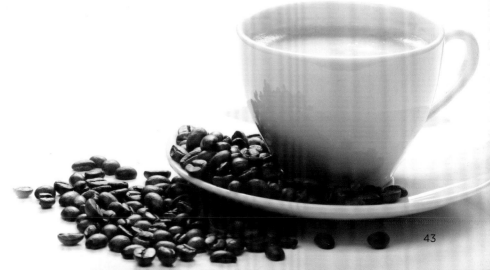

High mercury fish

Fish is a healthy part of any well-balanced diet and is especially important for pregnant women as it is rich in beneficial omega-3 fats. These fats are essential for the optimal growth and development of your baby's brain and nervous system. However, some types of fish contain high levels of heavy metals, namely mercury, which can affect your baby's health. Clearly, these should be avoided during pregnancy.

High levels of mercury can cause damage to a baby's nervous system and brain. Unborn babies are particularly vulnerable to the effects of mercury, due to their smaller size and developing nervous systems and brains. The foetus appears to be most sensitive to the effects of mercury during the third and fourth months of a pregnancy. Babies exposed to high levels of mercury in the womb may be left with attention, learning and memory problems.

Fish to avoid

Swordfish, shark (flake), tilefish, marlin, orange roughy (sea perch) and tuna (bluefin, albacore). Mercury levels in tuna can vary greatly based on the type and where it was caught. To be safe, pregnant women should avoid or severely limit their intake of tuna. Canned tuna is thought to have lower levels.

Best fish

Salmon (canned, fresh), trout, mackerel and sardines, anchovies, herring, cod (Alaskan), halibut (pacific and Atlantic) and haddock.

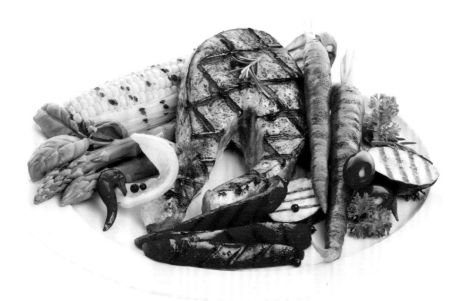

BPA - toxic 'hormone-mimicking' plastic chemicals

Bisphenol-A or BPA is a synthetic chemical compound used in the production of a variety of plastics, commonly found in water bottles, plastic containers, canned food linings and even some baby bottles.

This chemical has been found to act like an artificial oestrogen in the body, which can interfere with normal hormonal signalling and cause a number of health problems. Exposure in the womb to BPA can increase your child's chances of developing breast cancer as an adult, and contribute to the likelihood of them having wheezing problems in the first six months of life. [4]

BPA is also associated with reduced fertility and immune function, early puberty in children, and menstrual irregularities. Because their reproductive organs are still developing, unborn babies, infants and children are especially vulnerable to the effect of BPA. For this reason pregnant women should take care to avoid BPA contaminated products for their health and the health of their baby.

Taking folic acid when you're pregnant not only protects your baby from neural tube defects but may also help protect your baby from the effects of BPA.

Trace amounts of BPA can leach from plastic containers made with BPA into foods and drink. Ways to avoid ingesting BPAs include buying and storing foods in glass or stainless steel containers, using stainless steel or glass water bottles, and not heating food in plastic containers or with plastic cling wrap. Avoid buying plastic lined canned foods, especially foods that are acidic (tomatoes, citrus, soft drink). Buy BPA-free teething rings, dummies, baby bottles, and toys. Avoid plastic food containers and bottles with recycling label No. 7 or the letters "PC" on the bottom, as they contain BPAs. Trace amounts of BPA can leach from these containers into foods and drink. Plastics with the recycling label 1, 2 and 4 are a better choice as they are BPA-free.

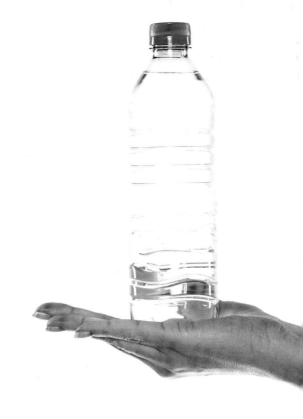

Safe and natural skin care

What you put on your skin during pregnancy can be just as important as what you put in your stomach. A good percentage of creams and cosmetics you put on your skin ends up in your blood stream. Pregnant women have to be particularly careful not to use any skin care products that contain potentially damaging chemicals that could affect their unborn baby's health. It's common for pregnant women to layer themselves in creams and oils to help prevent stretch marks, so it is important that they use something that is safe and natural.

As a rule of thumb, if you can't spell or pronounce an ingredient you can be pretty sure that it isn't natural, and if it's not safe enough for you and your baby to eat you shouldn't be putting it on your skin. Also, don't be fooled by labels that say 'natural', 'dermatological tested' or 'organic' - this doesn't mean it's chemical free and safe for you or your baby. Read ingredients carefully.

Tips for choosing safe skin care products

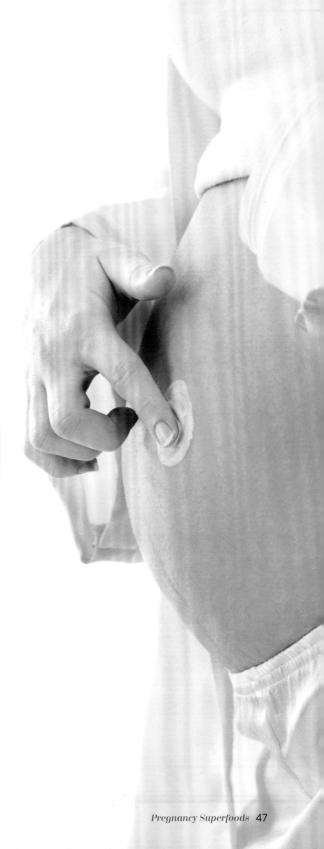

• Always choose 100% natural, preferably organic skin care products for you and your baby.

• Choose skin products made from natural sources such as cocoa butter, coconut oil, calendula oil, vitamin E, rose hip oil, apricot oil, almond oil, grape seed oil, jojoba oil, and wheat germ oil. These safe, natural ingredients will keep your skin well moisturised, nourished and hydrated, which will help prevent stretch marks and itchiness.

• Do not use creams containing mineral oils as they just coat the skin, giving the appearance and feeling of being moisturised. They actually inhibit the skin's ability to breath and absorb nutrients and moisture. Mineral oils make the skin think it's moisturised and in turn slows down its natural production of body oils. Mineral oil is what baby oil is made from, so refrain from using it on your baby too.

What are your cravings telling you?

Have you been craving some weird and wonderful things since you've fallen pregnant? Foods you would never normally eat?

Well this is perfectly normal and very common during pregnancy. Certain cravings however can indicate a possible nutritional deficiency, or it may be a consequence of having unbalanced blood sugar levels, and being fatigued.

Some of the more common food cravings include sugary foods, usually a sign that you have unstable blood sugar levels and that your energy levels are low. **Craving sweets** can also be an indication that you are deficient in the mineral chromium.

If **salty foods** have been more your thing lately and you have been tucking into chips, crackers and pickles, this could be a sign that your adrenal glands are fatigued and are under-functioning.

Chocolate cravings could be a reflection of a magnesium deficiency, or maybe you chasing that endorphin rush you get when chocolate hits your mouth?

Craving red meat could be a sign that you are low in iron or zinc, which are both important minerals during pregnancy, and both commonly deficient in expectant mums.

Cravings for milk, cheese and dairy foods is often associated with a calcium deficiency, or is the body's way of supplying your baby with plenty of this important bone-building mineral.

Some women crave **citrus fruits**, due to them having an acidic or metallic tasting saliva that can be relieved by eating citrus fruits such as lemons and grapefruit.

Some pregnant women have more bizarre cravings for non-food items like dirt, sand, chalk, soap or ice, this is called 'pica'. **Pica cravings** are thought to be associated with nutrient deficiencies. For example, craving ice can be a sign that you are low in iron. Giving in to most of these non-food cravings could be dangerous to you and your baby's health and should be resisted. Let your doctor, naturopath or nutritionist know, they will be able to help identify and eradicate the reasons for these cravings.

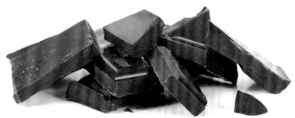

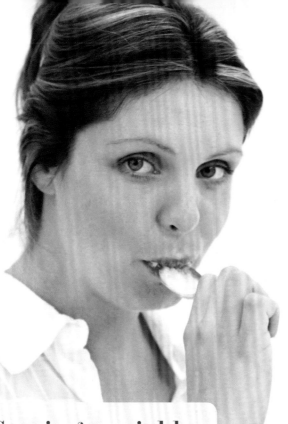

Cravings - pickles and ice cream anyone?

....

Pregnant women commonly get food cravings, some of which can be quite peculiar. Certain cravings can actually be the body's way of telling us that we're deficient in a certain vitamin or mineral, or that we have unbalanced blood sugar levels. Of course, a woman's taste and smell can change when she's pregnant and this would no doubt contribute to her different food choices. Pregnant women can come home with some weird and wonderful things after a grocery shop sometimes, food they would never normally eat.

Sugar cravings

During pregnancy you are prone to cravings that come in varying forms. Sometimes these are quite odd and completely out of character or may take the form of simple magnifications of normal temptations and partialities.

As is the case with most people, sugar cravings are common for expectant mums. However, during pregnancy, the implications of excessive sugar intake may be compounded.

Having sugar cravings is usually a sign that your blood sugar levels are unbalanced, and energy levels are low. When you lack energy - which of course is a common complaint during pregnancy – it is quite normal to crave sugary, carbohydrate foods so that blood sugar levels may rise again and provide a necessary energy boost.

It sounds obvious but the key to curbing sugar cravings is to take care to regulate your blood sugar levels; that is, to prevent dramatic spikes and drops in blood sugar. Not only will this reduce your desire to regularly consume foods with high sugar content, but it will also be of great benefit to the overall health of both mum and baby. Maintaining healthy blood sugar levels will help reduce the risk of gaining excessive weight during pregnancy and lower the risk of developing gestational diabetes, which can predispose your baby to type-2 diabetes later in life.

The following simple tips to help curb those dreaded sugar cravings, and give you the willpower to walk past the chocolate aisle next time you're in the supermarket, are simple but extremely effective.

Top tips for curbing sugar cravings

••••••••••••••••••••••••••••••••••••••

• Eat smaller, healthy meals and snacks more regularly, graze throughout the day.

• Don't skip meals, especially breakfast as it is the most important meal of the day. Skipping breakfast can set you up for a day of unstable blood sugar levels and poor food choices.

• Include protein-rich foods with each meal and with snacks. Protein helps stabilise blood sugar levels and curb sugar cravings. Some healthy protein choices include nuts and seeds, legumes, eggs, fish, lean meat and organic chicken, low-fat yoghurt and cheese, and soy products.

• Choose wholegrain carbohydrate foods over 'white', refined varieties. Wholegrains have a lower GI and are rich in dietary fibre. This has a balancing effect on blood sugar levels, slowing the absorption of glucose from foods eaten and reducing the sharp rise in blood sugar levels. Fibre-rich foods include whole oats, brown rice, quinoa, grainy breads, wholegrain pasta, legumes, fruits and vegetables.

• The mineral chromium is beneficial for normalising blood sugar levels and can really help dampen sugar cravings. You can increase your chromium intake by eating chromium-rich foods such as broccoli, wholegrain cereals, nuts, mushrooms and soy beans.

• Taking a magnesium supplement will also help to keep your blood sugar levels in check.

Raspberry leaf tea

Raspberry leaf (Rubus idaeus) is a safe and widely-used herb in pregnancy, commonly taken in the last trimester. Raspberry leaf helps to strengthen, tone and relax the muscles used for delivery, preparing you for childbirth. Using raspberry leaf in the last stages of pregnancy is thought to help reduce the pain and duration of labour and birth.

Another benefit of raspberry leaf is that it is extremely nourishing, a good source of a variety of essential nutrients such as vitamins A, B, C and E, and minerals iron, zinc, calcium, potassium and magnesium.

Raspberry leaf can also help ease morning sickness for some women and can be taken after the birth to help promote and enrich breast milk production.

Recommended dosage

Drink 1 – 2 cups a day during the second trimester and 3 – 4 cups a day during the third trimester.

Add 1 tsp of raspberry leaf tea or leaf tea or 1 teabag to a cup of boiling water and let it steep for 10 minutes, then drink. You can add lemon wedges or a little honey for taste if you wish.

If taking tablets start with 2 x 300mg or 400mg tablets 3 times a day during the last trimester.

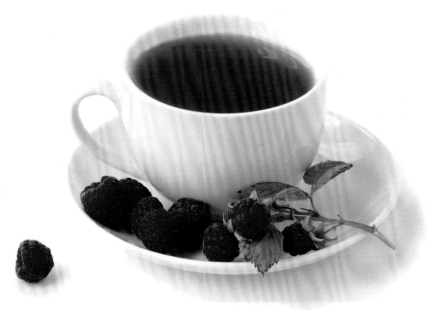

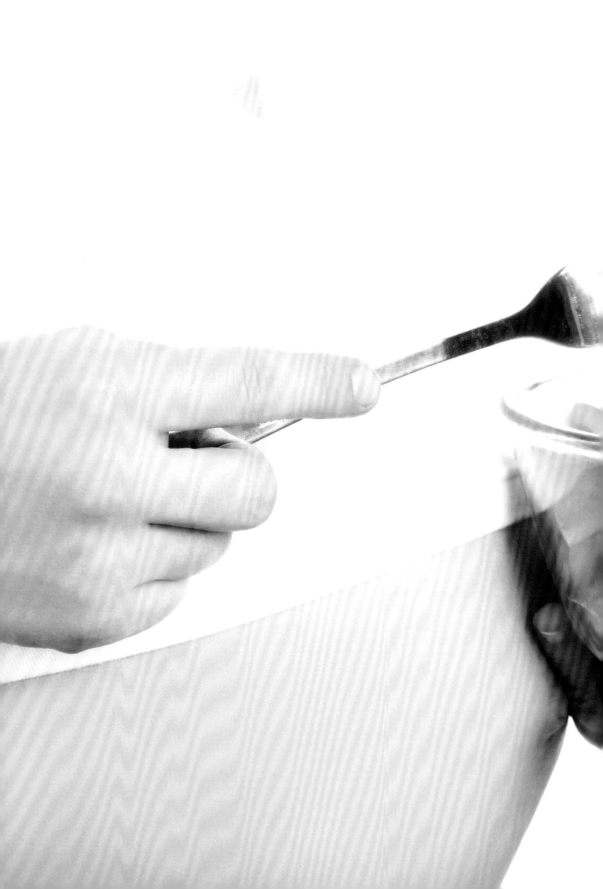

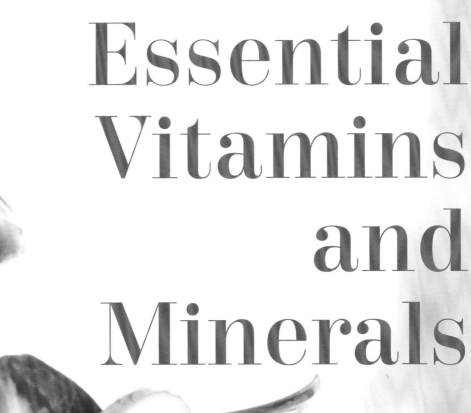

Essential Vitamins and Minerals

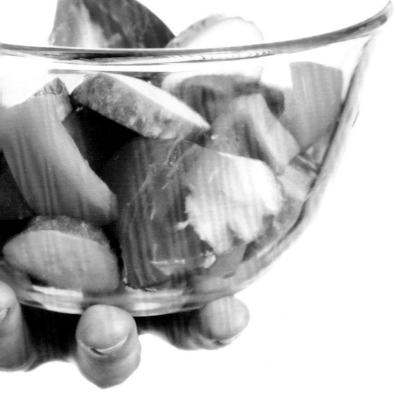

Vitamin A

(Retinol) & Beta-Carotene

Vitamin A is essential for your baby's growth and the development of their heart, lungs, kidneys and other important organs. Vitamin A also plays a role in the development of your baby's eyes and is needed to maintain healthy eyesight.

You and your baby need adequate levels of vitamin A to support proper immune function and keep your gut mucous membranes healthy, to protect you from infections.

Good vitamin A levels will also help women heal after birthing if there has been any tissue tearing. Deficiencies in vitamin A are associated with miscarriage and congenital abnormalities.

During pregnancy, it is important not to get too much vitamin A (retinol), as it can cause birth defects and liver toxicity in high doses. It is recommended that pregnant women do not exceed 3,000 mcg RAE (10,000 IU) of vitamin A daily, through supplementation and foods. The recommended dosage of vitamin A for pregnant women is around 770 mcg RAE of vitamin A (2,565 IU) daily and 1,300 mcg RAE (4,330 IU) while breastfeeding.

Beta-carotene, however, is a safer option for pregnant women and is converted to vitamin A in the body. You can't overdose on beta-carotene from vegetable and fruit sources. If you do have high levels in your diet you may notice the palms of your hands or soles of your feet go an orange colour, especially if you drink a lot of carrot juice. This isn't harmful to your health.

Best Food Sources

Vitamin A is found in animal products such as eggs, milk, meat, fish and fortified cereals. Beta-carotene is mainly found in red, yellow, orange and dark green fruits and vegetables, including carrots, apricots, pumpkin, red capsicum, tomatoes, spinach and kale.

B vitamins

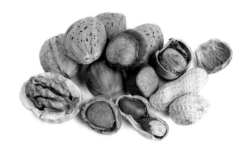

The B vitamins are a closely related group of vitamins that are vital for many important processes in the body and are particularly important during pregnancy when there is a higher demand for energy.

B vitamins act as 'anti-stress' vitamins, they are needed for a healthy functioning nervous system and are helpful during times of increased physical or emotional stress such as pregnancy.

A woman's blood volume increases by nearly 50% during pregnancy and B6 (Pyridoxine) is required to help make all those extra red blood cells. This B vitamin also helps maintain healthy blood sugar levels, is effective for treating morning sickness, and supports healthy immune function, which can easily be compromised during pregnancy.

Expectant mums should take a combination of all the B vitamins for a healthy pregnancy and a healthy baby. A quality pregnancy multi-vitamin should contain a good combination of your B vitamins.

Together with folic acid and vitamin B12, B6 helps maintain healthy homocysteine levels. If elevated levels of this substance are found, there may be an increased risk of heart disease and pregnancy complications such as preeclampsia (elevated blood pressure), recurrent pregnancy loss, and giving birth to a baby of low birth weight.

Best Food Sources

Foods rich in B vitamins include wholegrain cereals and bread, wheat germ, nuts, seeds, legumes, meat, poultry, salmon, eggs, milk and green leafy vegetables (a good source of folate).

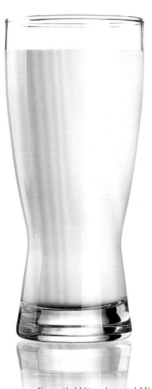

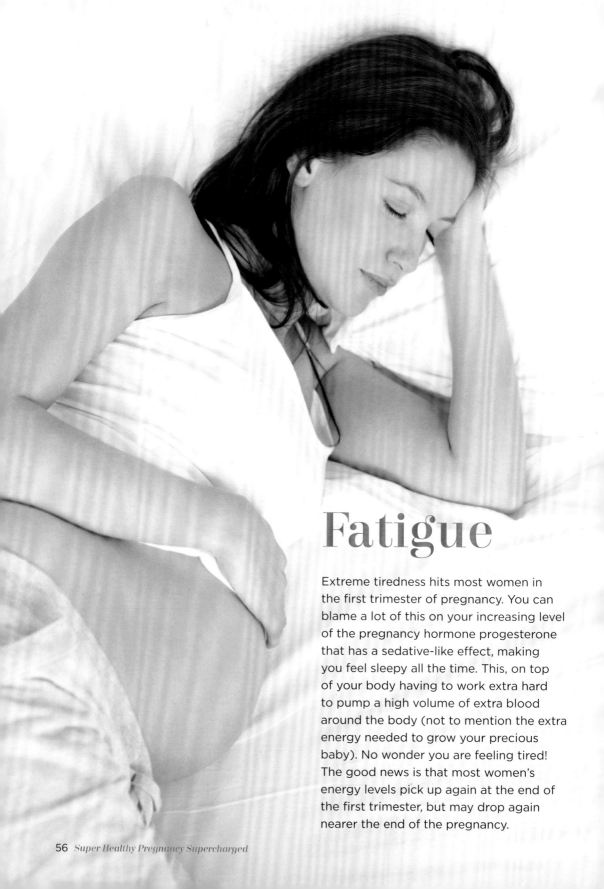

Fatigue

Extreme tiredness hits most women in the first trimester of pregnancy. You can blame a lot of this on your increasing level of the pregnancy hormone progesterone that has a sedative-like effect, making you feel sleepy all the time. This, on top of your body having to work extra hard to pump a high volume of extra blood around the body (not to mention the extra energy needed to grow your precious baby). No wonder you are feeling tired! The good news is that most women's energy levels pick up again at the end of the first trimester, but may drop again nearer the end of the pregnancy.

There are some things you can do however to give yourself a much needed boost in energy.

It's important to get plenty of sleep and go to bed earlier than usual to recharge your batteries. Have naps during the day if you can or even just put your feet up for a while with a herbal tea and a good book. The more sleep and rest you get the better.

It's important for pregnant women to eat a well-balanced diet rich in unprocessed, wholesome foods such as fruit, vegetables, legumes, nuts, seeds, and wholegrain cereals. A healthy diet is important to supply you (and your baby) with all the vitamins and minerals you need for energy production and good health. Drinking plenty of water is also important, aim for around 2 litres a day.

Keep your energy levels up by eating small, frequent meals throughout the day, including nutritious protein-rich snacks. Limit any sugary, processed foods that will cause your blood sugar levels to rise rapidly then plummet, which will leave you feeling even more exhausted. Protein-rich meals will help stabilise your blood sugar levels and help you maintain more balanced energy levels. Good protein choices include nuts, seeds, yoghurt, organic eggs and chicken, fish, lean meat, tofu and legumes (hummus).

Choose wholegrain, complex carbohydrate foods (wholegrain breads and pasta, brown rice, quinoa and whole oats), over refined 'white' carbohydrates (white bread and pasta, commercially baked cakes and cookies, sugary breakfast cereals).

B vitamins and magnesium are two important nutrients needed for energy production. Your pregnancy multi should contain good levels of B vitamins. You may want to add a magnesium supplement and increase magnesium and B vitamin rich foods in the diet such as wholegrain cereals, nuts, seeds, legumes, eggs, milk and green leafy vegetables.

Low iron levels are common in pregnancy and will cause low energy levels. Make sure you eat plenty of iron rich foods such as red meat, legumes and green leafy vegetables, and if you are tested deficient take an iron supplement.

Spirulina can help give you a boost in energy as it's an extremely nutrient-rich food and includes B vitamins, iron and magnesium. A good maintenance dose is 5 - 6 tablets or capsules a day. You can also get spirulina powder, but it does have a seaweed-like smell so if you're already feeling a little queasy then capsules are your best option.

Lighten your work load and delegate jobs around the home, and cut back on strenuous exercise; try walking, swimming and prenatal yoga instead. This can be very difficult if you're working full time in a busy job.

Vitamin B12
(Cyanocobalamin)

Vitamin B12 is another important B vitamin for pregnant women as it assists with the healthy growth and development of a baby's nervous system and brain. Mothers deficient in B12 may become fatigued and anaemic, and have a higher risk of having a baby with spinal cord damage.

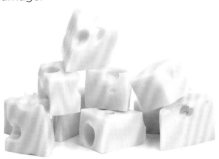

Best Food Sources

B12 is only found in animal products such as meat, poultry, fish, shellfish, eggs, milk, cheese and yoghurt, and fortified foods such as soy milk, yeast extracts and cereals. Our beneficial intestinal bacteria can also make B12.

Best Food Sources

The best sources of folate are dark green leafy vegetables (e.g. spinach, kale, turnip and mustard greens, parsley, collard greens, broccoli) and legumes such as lentils.

You can also buy folic acid fortified foods such as breads, cereals, flours, pasta, rice and other grain products.

Folic acid
(Folate)

Folic acid is a type of B vitamin that is the man-made synthetic form of folate, found in supplements and added to fortified foods. Folate is the natural form found in foods such as green leafy vegetables. We need a continuous supply of folate in our diet as our body cannot store it. This B vitamin is particularly important during pregnancy, where your daily recommended dosage doubles.

Good folate levels are essential for healthy foetal development and to help prevent neural tube defects such as spina bifida. It is recommended that pregnant women take 500-600mcg of folic acid daily throughout their pregnancy, and preferably start 3 months before conception.

Vitamin C

Good vitamin C levels during pregnancy are a must, as it fulfils so many important roles in keeping you and your baby healthy. Vitamin C, or ascorbic acid, acts as a highly effective antioxidant, protecting cells in the body from free radical damage. It also plays a significant role in the formation of collagen, which is a component of your growing baby's blood vessels, tendons, ligaments, bones, teeth and skin.

Vitamin C helps promote a healthy immune system too, which expectant mums need to fight off colds and infections. Vitamin C increases the absorption of essential pregnancy nutrients, iron and calcium, and helps to convert folic acid into its active form for the body to use.

Best Food Sources

Vitamin C-rich foods include citrus fruits, berries, rose hips, black currents, capsicum, papaya, chilli peppers, broccoli, kale, cabbage and spinach.

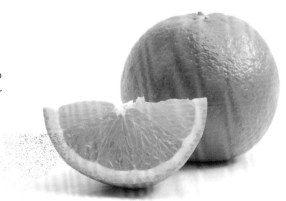

Bioflavonoids

Bioflavonoids, including rutin and hesperidin, are often found in vitamin C-rich foods, and work with vitamin C to enhance its activity. Bioflavonoids are important for protecting and preserving the structure and tone of capillaries and blood vessels, and are useful for preventing or reducing haemorrhoids and varicose veins in pregnancy.

Best Food Sources

Bioflavonoids can be found in red capsicum, berries, citrus fruits, broccoli, Brussels sprouts, green tea, garlic, onion and buckwheat.

Vitamin D

Vitamin D or "the sunshine vitamin" as it's known, is essential for your baby's optimal bone health. It increases calcium absorption and mineral deposition in bones, which promotes the growth and development of bones and teeth. Vitamin D is also heralded as having anti-cancer effects and is important for boosting immunity.

Low vitamin D levels in pregnancy are linked to insulin resistance and an increased risk of developing gestational diabetes. Vitamin D deficiency may also be associated with an increased risk of infant allergic rhinitis, asthma, type-1 diabetes, and autoimmune diseases. Ask your doctor to check your vitamin D levels early in your pregnancy. If your blood results come back low it is recommended that you start taking a vitamin D supplement at a dosage of 1000iu daily. Taking a vitamin D supplement during pregnancy and after will also help protect women against osteoporosis later on in life.

Best Food Sources

Sunlight is the easiest and healthiest way to get sufficient vitamin D. Vitamin D is found in oily fish (salmon, trout, mackerel, and sardines) and eggs. Milk such as cow's, soy and rice are fortified with vitamin D. Cod liver oil is also a good source, however it is not recommended in pregnancy due to its high vitamin A levels.

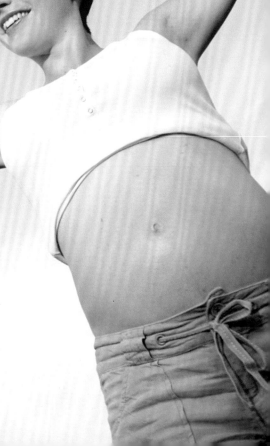

Vitamin E

Your baby needs a good supply of vitamin E to nourish and support their developing nervous system. Babies born with a deficiency may develop neurological problems. Newborn infants, especially premature infants, are vulnerable to vitamin E deficiency because they have low tissue reserves. Mothers pass on around 20mg of vitamin E to their baby in the last 12 weeks of pregnancy.

Vitamin E is another potent antioxidant that helps fight free radical damage in the body and helps prevent illness. Good levels of vitamin E will also help reduce the risk of high blood pressure, which is commonly seen in pregnancy.

Best Food Sources

Foods rich in vitamin E include cold pressed olive oil, sunflower oil, safflower oil, wheat germ, wholegrain cereals, green leafy vegetables, avocado, fish, eggs and raw nuts and seeds (sunflower, pumpkin, sesame).

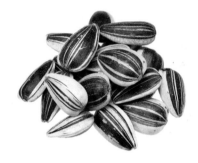

Best Food Sources

We get vitamin K from foods such as green leafy vegetables, cauliflower, dairy products, soy beans and eggs. The majority of our vitamin K is produced in the body by beneficial bowel bacteria. If your bowel flora is compromised through taking antibiotics or poor diet, it will interfere with your vitamin K production.

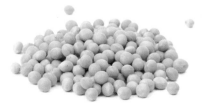

Vitamin K

Vitamin K is essential for normal blood clotting, and is essential for preventing and controlling excessive bleeding.

A deficiency in vitamin K during pregnancy could increase the risk of heavy bleeding after birth. Vitamin K also plays a role in building strong, healthy bones.

Babies are generally born with lower vitamin K levels. Newborn are routinely given vitamin K injections soon after birth, especially if it has been a difficult birth, to reduce the risk of bleeding in the brain. Vitamin K can also be given to babies orally. Talk to your doctor or midwife about your options.

Zinc

Zinc would have to be one of the most important minerals during pregnancy. Pregnant women need a good supply of this super mineral to sustain a healthy pregnancy and to support the optimal growth and development of their baby.

Worried about stretch marks? Zinc is your friend; needed for the proper formation of elastin in connective tissue, which helps prevent stretch marks, perineal tears during the birth and cracked nipples when breastfeeding. Zinc is also necessary for healthy growth and development of your baby's skeletal muscles and bones, and is required for healthy immune function and brain formation.

The case for dietary zinc is clear when you consider that low zinc status is associated with low birth weight babies, premature delivery, and even congenital malformations that have been linked to SIDS. Low zinc levels (and high copper levels) after birth can contribute to post natal depression.

A majority of pregnant women are unfortunately deficient in this important mineral yet your zinc levels can easily be tested using the zinc taste test by your naturopath or at your local health food store. If your levels are low, supplementation is recommended at a dosage of around 50mg a day. Liquid zinc supplements are easily absorbed and are very effective for bringing zinc levels up quickly. Make sure you take zinc supplements after food as it can make you feel nauseous on an empty stomach.

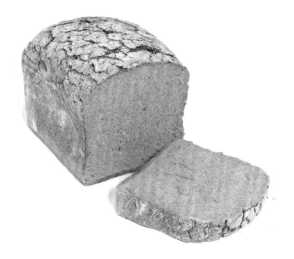

Best Food Sources

Zinc is found in a wide variety of foods. The best food sources include lean meat, chicken, fish, milk, cheese and other dairy foods, eggs (yolks), legumes (soy beans, lima beans, lentils, peas), wholegrain cereals and breads, sunflower and pumpkin seeds, and pecans. Zinc is lost during the refining of grains, so always choose wholegrain varieties.

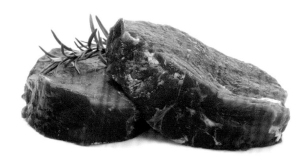

Calcium

Optimal calcium levels are crucial for your baby's teeth and bone development.

Rapid skeletal growth begins in the second trimester and continues right throughout the pregnancy. Your baby will draw on your own calcium reserves if you are not getting enough calcium. It is important that all expectant mums have a good supply of calcium in their diets and through supplementation to reduce the risk the depletion of their own bone and teeth health, which could lead to dental problems and osteoporosis later in life.

Adequate calcium levels will also help pregnant women maintain normal blood pressure, reduce fluid retention, and reduce the risk of pregnancy-induced hypertension and preeclampsia.

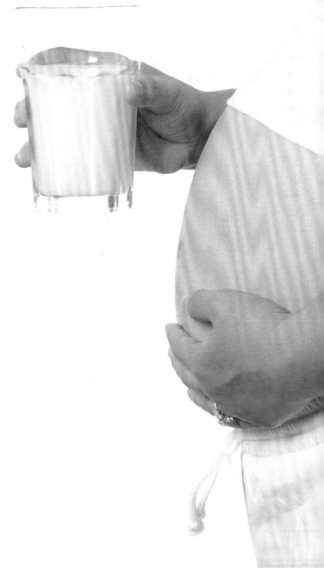

Best Food Sources

Foods rich in calcium include milk and other dairy products such as cheese and yoghurt, nuts (especially almonds), sunflower and sesame seeds (tahini), the bones of tinned fish (salmon, sardines), tofu, calcium fortified soy and rice milks, and green leafy vegetables.

Iron

Iron is a very important mineral for pregnant women as it is needed to make red blood cells. During pregnancy a woman's blood volume increases by nearly half, which increases her iron requirements significantly. Iron is needed for haemoglobin production, the portion of red blood cells that transport oxygen around you and your baby's body.

Iron is also needed for proper immune function, and for healthy formation of your baby's brain, eyes and bones.

Low iron levels will leave you feeling tired and worn out, and more vulnerable to colds, flu and other illnesses. You especially don't want to be low in iron after the birth, you will need all the energy you can get to manage running on minimal sleep.

Iron deficiency is a common cause of anaemia (low red blood cell count) and is associated with a higher risk of pre-term delivery and subsequent low birth weight. Your baby will be born with a stored supply of iron, which will last around 6 months. If you are deficient in iron during pregnancy this can affect your baby's iron stores.

Best Food Sources

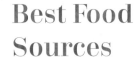

You will find plenty of iron in red meat, chicken, fish and eggs, as well as legumes, nuts, seeds, green leafy vegetables, wheat germ, and soy products.

Your doctor will test your iron levels throughout your pregnancy, as it is common for deficiencies to occur especially in the second and third trimester when your blood volume increases dramatically.

This increased need for iron cannot always be met by the diet alone so supplementation in pregnancy is often recommended. A preventative dose of 30mg of elemental iron daily is recommended. Women who have been diagnosed with low iron levels should take around 50mg of elemental iron daily, and increase iron-rich foods in their diet. Some over-the-counter iron medications cause constipation, which you are trying to avoid during pregnancy. Ask your local naturopath or nutritionist for a good iron supplement that won't cause this uncomfortable side effect.

Tip

To increase iron absorption, include vitamin C-rich foods with your meal. For example, have a drink of orange juice, water with fresh lemon or a tomato based sauce with a meal. Drinking tea, coffee or soft drink with a meal will actually inhibit iron absorption.

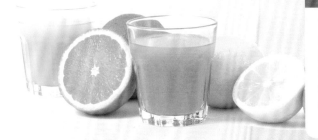

Iron Deficiency and Anaemia

Women produce nearly 50% more blood than usual while they are pregnant, which also considerably increases their need for iron. Iron is essential for haemoglobin production, which is the protein in red blood cells that have the job of transporting oxygen to every cell in your body and to your baby.

Iron is an important mineral for your baby's growth and development. It is needed to build a healthy immune system, for the production of white blood cells and antibodies, and is required for baby's brain development and function.

Your doctor will test your iron levels during your first antenatal appointment, and again in your second trimester. A lot of women's iron levels drop in pregnancy, especially in the second and third trimester when the amount of blood in your body increases dramatically, which can result in anaemia (low red blood cell count).

Babies are born with a supply of iron, which usually lasts them around 6 months. If your iron levels are low in pregnancy your baby's iron stores may be compromised, which can increase their susceptibility to infections and anaemia later in infancy.

Common symptoms of iron deficiency and anaemia include tiredness, dizziness, pale skin and lowered immune function. Inadequate iron levels can also leave mothers feeling fatigued and washed out after the birth. Iron-deficiency anaemia during pregnancy is linked to an increased risk of preterm delivery and low birth weight, and may increase your risk of postnatal depression.

How to prevent iron deficiency and anaemia:

• Of course it is important for pregnant women to eat a healthy, well-balanced diet including iron-rich foods. However, it can be difficult for pregnant women to get sufficient iron through foods alone so supplementation is recommended to meet your increasing needs. It is recommended that pregnant women take an iron supplement with 30mg of elemental iron daily, as a preventative measure, and 50mg a day if you have been diagnosed with an iron deficiency. Most over the counter iron supplements cause constipation, which is common in pregnancy. If this is the case ask your local naturopath or nutritionist for an iron supplement that won't cause constipation.

• Calcium can interfere with absorption so make sure you take iron supplements away from calcium supplements, and don't wash them down with milk. Coffee and tea can also hinder absorption, due to them containing polyphenols.

• Include plenty of iron-rich foods in your diet including lean meat, chicken, fish and eggs, wholegrain cereals, wheat germ, legumes, nuts, seeds, green leafy vegetables, dried fruits (dates, prunes, apricots), and iron-fortified cereals.

• You can increase iron absorption by having foods rich in vitamin C with a meal, e.g. orange juice, water with fresh lemon, tomato based sauce, berries, broccoli or cabbage.

Magnesium

Expectant mums need appropriate levels of magnesium to help prevent leg cramps, minimise fluid retention and help ease morning sickness, all of which are common pregnancy complaints. Magnesium also plays a role in regulating blood sugar levels and blood pressure, which will help reduce the risk of gestational diabetes and pre-eclampsia.

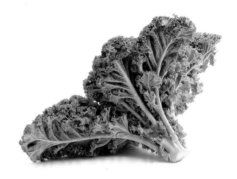

Magnesium is the perfect supplement for tired and stressed expectant mums. Magnesium is required to produce energy in the body, but is also considered the 'anti-stress' mineral as it supports healthy nervous system function, relieves anxiety and helps you sleep more soundly. Your baby also needs a good supply of magnesium for the development of their bones, teeth and nervous system.

Best Food Sources

Good sources of magnesium include pumpkin seeds, sunflower seeds, wheat germ, yoghurt, tofu, nuts (almonds, cashews), cocoa, mineral water, parsnips, soy beans, tofu, green leafy vegetables, wholegrain cereals and seaweed.

Another benefit of magnesium for expectant mums is that it helps make the perineum stretchier, and good levels during labor ensures that the uterus contracts effectively and the cervix dilates easily. Magnesium supplementation during pregnancy has been shown to help prevent premature uterine contractions.

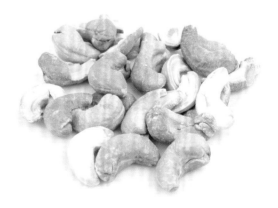

A magnesium deficiency during pregnancy has been associated with an increased risk of miscarriage, developmental problems, low birth weight, and pre-eclampsia (a serious condition which results in high blood pressure and swelling of the hands, feet and face).

Tips for easing or preventing fluid retention

....

• Fluid retention is not a sign that you've been drinking too much water, so continue to drink plenty of water throughout the day.

• Reduce your salt intake by limiting processed, canned and fast foods that are commonly high in sodium. Excessive salt in the diet will promote fluid retention.

• Magnesium is an important mineral that helps regulate water balance in the body. Magnesium supplementation can be very beneficial for preventing fluid retention. Foods rich in magnesium include nuts, seeds, legumes, green leafy vegetables and wholegrain cereals.

• Vitamin B6 also helps control water balance in the body and can be useful for easing fluid retention. The richest sources of vitamin B6 include fish, brown rice, garlic, kale, green beans, spinach, broccoli, and sunflower and sesame seeds.

• Fluid retention is generally worse by the end of the day, if you've been on your feet too long or in hot weather. Try to stay cool, don't spend long periods on your feet, put your feet up and rest when you can. Flying on planes can also cause your legs to swell, so support stockings can be helpful. Wearing comfortable flat shoes is also recommended.

Magnesium is an important mineral that helps regulate water balance in the body.

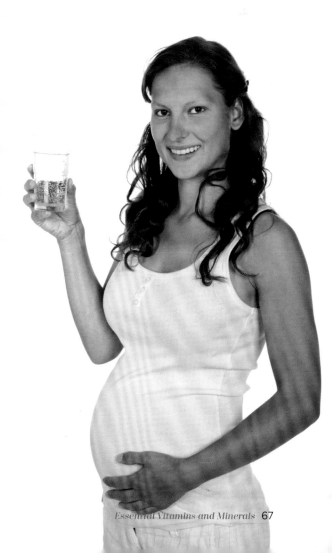

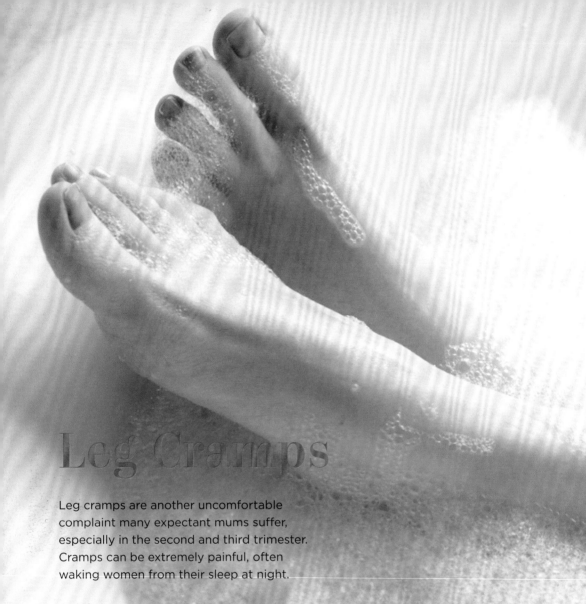

Leg Cramps

Leg cramps are another uncomfortable complaint many expectant mums suffer, especially in the second and third trimester. Cramps can be extremely painful, often waking women from their sleep at night.

A deficiency in either magnesium or calcium can cause leg cramps. These minerals play a major role in stimulating nerves and muscles to contract and relax properly. The weight of your growing baby putting pressure on your pelvic region and legs, slowing down circulation, is another contributing factor. Mums-to-be that put on a lot of weight quickly or who are carrying twins may be more prone to leg cramps. For preventing cramps, take around 400 – 600mg of magnesium and 1,500mg of calcium daily.

A nice warm bath at the end of the day can help relax and soothe sore muscles.

Tips for preventing or relieving muscle cramps

....

• Taking a calcium and magnesium supplement can be extremely beneficial for preventing cramps. You want to take around 400 – 600mg of magnesium and 1,500mg of calcium daily.

• Do not stand or sit with your legs crossed for long periods, this will reduce the circulation to your legs. If you get a cramp, stretch your legs and flex your feet upward, then massage the cramping area, or walk around until it stops.

• Doing regular gentle forms of exercise like swimming, walking and prenatal yoga will help reduce cramping. Doing calf and leg stretches daily can also be beneficial. Doing these before bed is recommended if you are prone to leg cramps while sleeping.

• A nice warm bath at the end of the day can help relax and soothe sore muscles.

• Drink plenty of water as dehydration can also cause muscle cramps.

• If you have a constant pain in your legs, along with swelling, call your doctor to rule out any serious conditions such as blood clotting in the leg vein (venous thromboembolism). Though this condition is very rare, it is better to be safe and have it checked out.

Selenium

Selenium is one of our major natural antioxidants, which helps support healthy thyroid function and immunity. Selenium can also help pregnant women maintain healthy blood pressure, and plays an active role in protecting against environmental pollutants. Although pregnant women have a greater need for selenium, they can usually get all the selenium they need through a healthy, well-balanced diet. Selenium in large amounts, over 400mcg per day, especially in pregnancy, can be toxic, so always read nutritional supplement labels for selenium and avoid in pregnancy.

The recommended dietary allowance of selenium for pregnant women is between 60-200mcg per day. Do not exceed 400mcg of selenium per day.

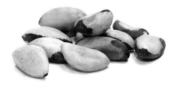

Best Food Sources

Brazil nuts are one of the best sources and just 2 will give you your daily recommended dose of selenium.

Other good sources include wholegrains (wheat, oats, corn, and rice) and legumes.

Chromium

Chromium is an important mineral during pregnancy as it helps maintain healthy blood sugar levels, and can help reduce sugar cravings and the risk of gestational diabetes. Your baby needs chromium to promote the building of proteins and tissues in their body.

Pregnant women require around 30mcg of chromium a day, and breastfeeding mothers 45 mcg a day.

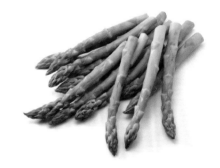

Best Food Sources

Foods rich in chromium include brewer's yeast, wholegrain breads and cereals, lean meat, cheese, prunes, asparagus, nuts and spinach.

One tablespoon of brewer's yeast contains 60 mcg of chromium, and 1 tablespoon of natural peanut butter contains 41 mcg.

Iodine

Iodine is a very important trace mineral that is needed for proper thyroid function, and is essential for your baby's nervous tissue and brain development.

Iodine is also important throughout childhood for normal growth and development, and healthy brain function. Even a mild iodine deficiency can lower a child's IQ.

Research has shown that many pregnant women are unfortunately iodine deficient. Lack of iodine can cause hypothyroidism (goiter), and can be damaging to your baby's developing brain, resulting in intellectual disabilities and growth retardation. Low iodine levels have also been associated with miscarriage.

Best Food Sources

Kelp is one of richest sources of naturally occurring iodine. Kelp is easy to add into your daily diet and is used to make sushi, soups, salads and stir-fries. Alternatively, sprinkle powdered kelp in juice or over vegetables.

Other foods that are good sources of iodine include spirulina, seaweed, and seafood, dairy products, iodised salt, lima beans, mushrooms, and sunflower seeds. Increasing salt to increase your iodine levels is not recommended, especially in pregnancy as it will promote fluid retention.

Potassium

Good levels of potassium are essential for a healthy pregnancy and baby. Potassium plays an important role in maintaining electrolyte and fluid balance in the body. Potassium helps keep blood pressure in check. During pregnancy women produce nearly 50% more blood volume, which requires extra potassium (and other electrolytes) to keep this extra fluid in the correct chemical balance.

Potassium is required for healthy nerve and muscle function as well as building muscle and for optimal growth.

A deficiency in potassium can be a result of chronic vomiting in pregnancy or diarrhoea, or from a poor diet. Pregnant women who get leg cramps in the middle of the night may be low in potassium (or calcium and magnesium).

Pregnant women should be having around 4,700mg of potassium a day, and 5,100mg a day when breastfeeding.

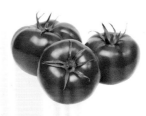

Best Food Sources

Fruits and vegetables (such as potato, cabbage, apricots, oranges, strawberries, bananas, avocado and tomato), nuts, seeds, soy products, red meat, chicken, fish, yoghurt and milk all provide potassium.

Importance of nutritional supplementation during pregnancy

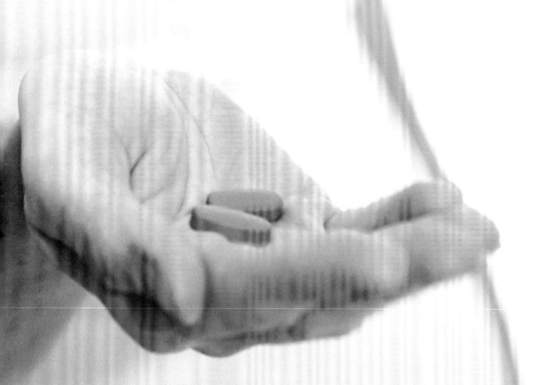

Although nothing takes away from the importance of a healthy, well-balanced diet, nutritional supplementation during pregnancy is extremely important. Even with the best intentions it can be hard to meet all of your nutritional needs during pregnancy with diet alone, when your intake needs double.

Taking specific nutritional supplements during pregnancy is like an insurance policy, making sure you are getting optimal levels of all the essential nutrients you need to sustain a healthy pregnancy and meet the nutritional demands of your growing baby. Your body must have a sufficient supply of these nutrients present at all times otherwise it could impact your baby's health.

Recommended nutritional supplements for expectant mums

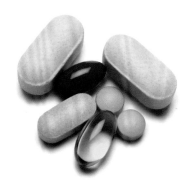

PREGNANCY MULTI-VITAMIN
(with 500mcg of folic acid)

Good quality **FISH OIL**
(2 x 1,000mg capsules daily)

VITAMIN C
(2,000mg daily)

PROBIOTIC SUPPLEMENT
(especially important in last
trimester)

IRON
(30mg a day as a maintenance dose,
or 50mg of elemental iron a day
if tested deficient)

VITAMIN D3
(if tested deficient take 1,000iu
daily)

CALCIUM
(if intake of calcium-rich foods
are low, particularly helpful from
second trimester onwards when
bones are developing, take around
1,000-1,500mg of elemental
calcium daily)

MAGNESIUM
(for leg cramps, fluid retention, or
sugar cravings 400-600mg daily)

Supplementing with specific nutrients in pregnancy is known to help prevent congenital defects and malformations, which are often caused by nutritional deficiencies. Some nutritional deficiencies before pregnancy can easily go unnoticed; however they can severely compromise the development of your baby.

During pregnancy, significant nutrient donations are made to your growing baby, often resulting in the mother becoming deficient. This can leave her feeling exhausted, run-down and more susceptible to illness and postnatal complications, such as breastfeeding problems, postnatal depression and poor recovery after the birth.

Another good reason why pregnant women should augment their diets with nutritional supplements is because commercially grown foods just don't have the nutritional levels they used to, due to nutrient poor soil. Processing and some cooking methods only further deplete the nutrient content of our food, so it is recommended to eat organic produce whenever you can and use healthy cooking methods such as light steaming and baking.

Vital macronutrients in pregnancy

Protein - the building blocks of life

We've all heard the saying that proteins are the building blocks of life. Indeed, just as adequate dietary protein fuels your own ability to cope with pregnancy demands - for repairing fatigued tissues and stressed muscles - your baby's own growth is highly dependent upon you having a good supply of quality protein in your diet. This helps baby achieve appropriate growth and developmental milestones and, ultimately, an optimal birth weight.

Protein foods are broken down into amino acids, which your baby uses to build all the proteins in its body including bones, internal organs, blood, muscles, skin, hair and nails.

It is during the second trimester when your baby starts to grow rapidly that you need to increase your food intake to meet your baby's extra nutritional needs, and the best way to do this is by introducing a couple of extra protein-rich snacks into your daily diet. Some simple yet ultra-healthy protein snacks include mixed nuts and seeds with sun-dried fruit, tubs of yoghurt, hummus and vegetable sticks or wholegrain crackers, cottage cheese on rice cakes, a boiled egg, or almond butter on toasted fruit and nut loaf.

There is another critical reason why extra protein is essential for your health during pregnancy. Your blood volume increases significantly during pregnancy as you give life to the little person that is growing inside of you. This extra blood volume brings with it a need for a greater number of red blood cells, all of which are made from a number of different proteins. Increased dietary proteins are thus needed to make all of these extra red blood cells.

You also need protein to help heal and repair your body, which is especially important after the birth, to help support collagen production and prevent stretch marks, to reduce hair loss after the birth, and for optimal breast milk production.

Women whose diets are deficient in protein during pregnancy have a higher risk of having a low-birth weight baby. Making sure you are eating enough protein will also lower your risk of pre-eclampsia during pregnancy, and help keep blood sugar levels balanced, which will help reduce the risk of gestational diabetes.

How much protein should I be having?

Pregnant women should aim to increase their protein intake by 20 – 30g in the second trimester. Most people have on average around 60g of protein daily; pregnant women should aim to eat around 80 – 90g of protein daily.

You will get around 20g of protein from each of the following:
1 cup firm tofu, 5 tbsp natural peanut butter, 1 ½ cups cooked legumes, 2 cups yoghurt, 3 eggs, ½ cup cow's milk, 85g chicken, lamb, salmon or cheese.

Best Food Sources

You should try to get your protein from a variety of sources, vegetarian and animal based, such as fish, organic chicken and eggs, lean meat, legumes, tofu and other soy products, nuts, seeds and yoghurt, cheese and other dairy products, and seaweed and spirulina.

Good Fats
- omega-3s are baby's brain food

Did you know that you can improve your baby's brain development by eating certain types of good fats?

Omega-3 essential fatty acids, namely DHA (docosaheaenoic acid) are vital for your baby's brain and nervous system development and retina formation. These essential fats, which cannot be made in the body and have to be obtained through the diet, are the building blocks of your baby's brain. DHA is especially vital during the third trimester when your baby's brain is developing rapidly.

Good levels of DHA in pregnancy will enhance your baby's cognitive and intellectual ability in childhood, as well as reduce the risk of your child developing learning disabilities and behavioural problems such as ADHD.

Omega-3 fats are also extremely important for expectant mum's health. They help keep skin soft and supple, and reduce the likelihood of stretch marks, as well as support healthy immune function and circulation.

Women who are deficient in omega-3s during pregnancy are at a greater risk of suffering from pre-eclampsia, low birth weight and preterm labour, and postpartum depression.

The best food sources of omega-3 fats are oily fish (salmon, trout, mackerel and sardines), some nuts and seeds and their oils (chia and flax seeds, and walnuts). A good quality fish oil supplement is recommended during pregnancy to ensure you and your baby are getting optimal levels of this essential fat.

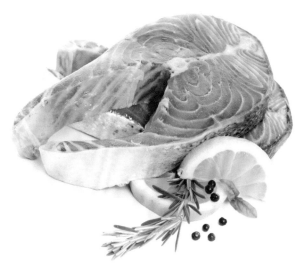

Enhance your baby's cognitive and intellectual ability in childhood.

Tips for preventing or reducing stretch marks

....

• Include plenty of foods rich in good fats, especially your omega-3 fats. These fats help keep the skin moist, soft and supple to help keep your skin elastic and less likely to tear as you grow bigger. The best sources of omega-3 fats are oily fish (salmon, trout, mackerel, and sardines), and flax and chia seeds and oil.

• A fish oil supplement is also recommended to increase your omega-3 intake. You should be taking a good quality fish oil supplement anyway throughout your pregnancy as it's important for your baby's brain and nervous system development and function. Take around 2-3g of omega-3s daily.

• Zinc and vitamin C are essential for collagen production, and are needed for tissue healing and cell growth and regeneration. Supplementation is recommended, so take around 2g of vitamin C and 45mg of zinc daily. Also include foods that are rich in zinc such as lean red meats, fish and chicken, yoghurt, cheese, sunflower and pumpkin seeds. Good sources of vitamin C include citrus fruits, berries, parsley, cabbage and broccoli.

• Drink plenty of water to make sure your skin is supple and well hydrated. Aim to drink around 1½ – 2 litres of water a day.

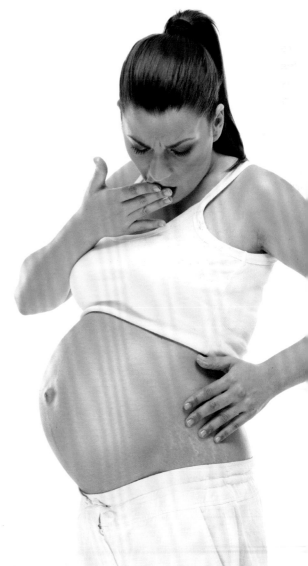

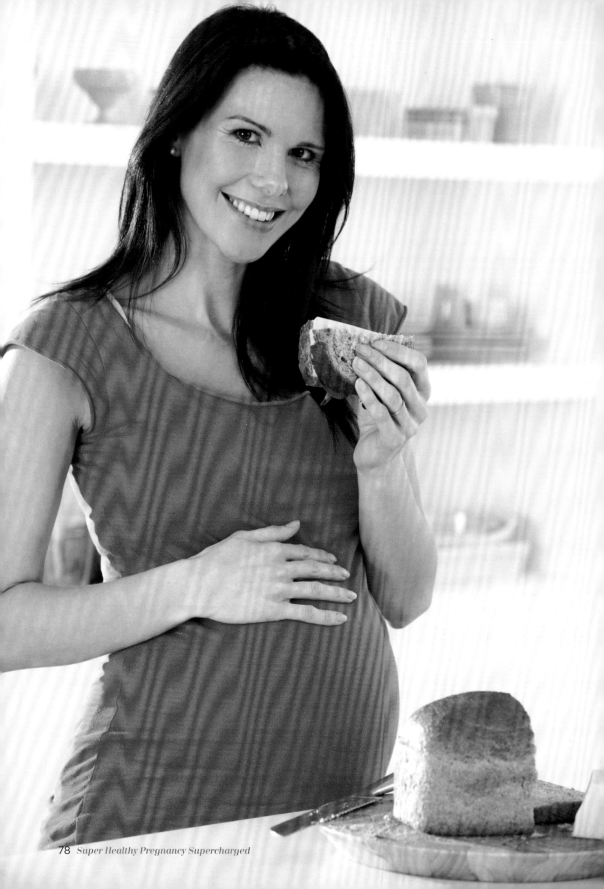

Wholegrains
– energy and fibre

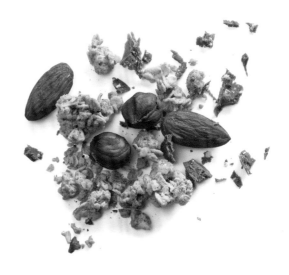

During pregnancy you need all the energy you can get and one of the best ways to do this is by eating wholesome wholegrain cereals such as brown rice, whole oats and muesli, quinoa, grainy breads and wholegrain crackers.

Wholegrains are an important part of any healthy, well-balanced diet. They're rich in complex carbohydrates, which will provide you with a slow and steady supply of glucose to fuel your brain and body. Your growing baby also needs plenty of energy to support their rapid growth and development.

Wholegrains are also your best source of dietary fibre, which pregnant women need to keep regular and to prevent constipation and haemorrhoids.

Due to wholegrains being high in fibre they are digested slower, which won't cause a sharp rise in blood sugar levels or spike in insulin. Wholegrains are also naturally rich in important pregnancy nutrients such as magnesium, selenium, potassium, B vitamins, zinc, iron and vitamin E. Choosing wholegrains over refined 'white' carbohydrate foods will also reduce excessive weight gain during pregnancy and the risk of gestational diabetes.

Wholegrains are naturally rich in important pregnancy nutrients such as magnesium, selenium, potassium, B vitamins, zinc, iron and vitamin E.

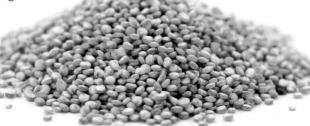

Fruits and Vegetables
- antioxidants and vitamins

Jam-packed with nutritional goodness, fruits and vegetables are an extremely important part of any pregnant woman's diet. They're rich in essential nutrients that expectant mums and their babies need for good health and optimal growth and development. These include vitamin C, for baby's collagen production and for healthy immune function; beta-carotene for healthy eyesight, and folic acid, needed to prevent neural tube defects. Fruits and vegetables also provide the minerals potassium and magnesium, which will help keep your blood pressure in check, and iron, which is needed in good amounts during pregnancy to make all of those extra red blood cells to nourish your baby.

The high fibre content of fruits and vegetables provides expectant mums with a number of health benefits such as preventing constipation and haemorrhoids, and helping keep blood sugar levels balanced to reduce the risk of gestational diabetes.

It is important to have a variety of different colours and types of fruits and vegetables in your diet as they all provide varying levels of essential vitamins, mineral and antioxidants. Eating a rainbow of colours will help maximise their nutritional benefits. For example, red and purple indicates the presence of a powerful antioxidant called anthocynanin, orange is rich in beta-carotene, and green and leafy contains plenty of iron and folate.

Brassica vegetables are also very important, such as broccoli, cauliflower and cabbage, as they are rich in cancer fighting and liver detoxing sulphur compounds. Root vegetables and legumes contain complex carbohydrates, which provide plenty of sustained energy, and legumes are an excellent source of protein to support your baby's rapid growth.

Fruits and vegetables are also high in fibre, which means they're digested slowly and help keep blood sugar levels stable, as well as keeping expectant mums regular and free from constipation and haemorrhoids.

Antioxidants
- optimise your and your baby's health

Antioxidants play a crucial part in maintaining a successful pregnancy and optimising the health and well-being of both baby and mother, but it also places an increased demand on your antioxidant supply.

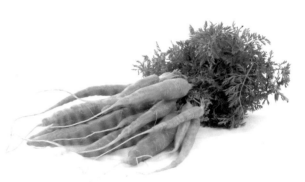

A number of nutrients act as antioxidants, which include selenium, zinc, vitamin E, beta-carotene and vitamins A and C. Antioxidants neutralise free radicals that can cause damage to cells in both the mother and baby. Free radicals are generated through normal metabolism and during normal placental development. If the mother hasn't got a good supply of antioxidants through supplementation and a good diet, free radicals can build up in the placenta and the mother's circulation, which could potentially result in adverse pregnancy outcomes.

Deficiencies of specific antioxidant nutrients, including selenium and zinc, can result in poor foetal growth, preeclampsia and the associated increased risk of diseases in adulthood such as cardiovascular disease and type 2 diabetes. [5]

Free radicals are also produced from stress, poor diet, smoking, alcohol, environmental pollution and excessive sun exposure. Antioxidants taken in combination may provide greater benefit than any single nutrient on its own.

According to a study out of The Children's Hospital of Philadelphia, women who consume high amounts of antioxidants before and during their pregnancies may be protecting their children against diabetes and obesity. [6]

Foods rich in antioxidants include berries (especially purple berries such as acai berries), purple, red and orange fruits and vegetables (tomatoes, red capsicum, beetroot, watermelon, carrots, pumpkin, red grapes) and citrus fruits.

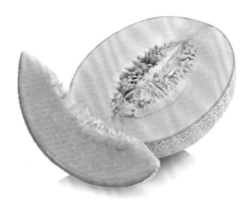

Probiotics

– good gut health means a strong immune system

We've all heard that yoghurt is good for us because it contains friendly bacteria that helps improve our digestion. But did you know just how important these friendly bacteria are for a pregnant woman and what role they play in your baby's future health?

Probiotic supplements and foods contain friendly bacteria, including lactobacillus, acidophilus and bifidus, which help promote a healthy balance of good bacteria in your intestines. A number of well-known fermented foods contain friendly bacteria, including yoghurt, fermented cheese, miso, tempeh, kefir and sauerkraut (fermented cabbage).

A balance of good intestinal bacteria is extremely important for promoting health and is needed for a healthy pregnancy and baby. Beneficial intestinal bacteria play a major role in your digestion, and for producing vitamins B12 and K, two vitamins that are important for your baby's nervous system development and for healthy blood clotting. Our immune function is also very dependent on a healthy balance of intestinal bacteria.

Taking a probiotic supplement during pregnancy and including probiotic-rich foods in the diet is an effective way for pregnant women to boost their immune system, and help treat or prevent

common complaints such as digestive problems, urinary tract infections, candida, and for restoring gut flora after antibiotic therapy.

Boosting your probiotic intake in pregnancy will also greatly benefit your baby's health. When a baby is in the womb its intestinal tract is sterile. Only after they are born are they exposed to many different species of microorganisms, which help set up their intestinal bacteria.

The main ways bacteria enter your baby's gut is when they come through the birth canal and swallow vaginal fluids, then from contact with people and from the surrounding environment. It is important during pregnancy that the mother has a healthy balance of good intestinal bacteria, as their intestinal health will affect the health of their baby.

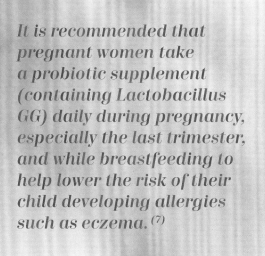

It is recommended that pregnant women take a probiotic supplement (containing Lactobacillus GG) daily during pregnancy, especially the last trimester, and while breastfeeding to help lower the risk of their child developing allergies such as eczema. [7]

Babies with poor intestinal health, who are lacking good levels of these beneficial bacteria, will have a greater risk of developing allergies in childhood such as eczema, asthma, hayfever, food allergies and intolerances. These babies will also have compromised immune health, becoming more vulnerable to catching colds, ear infections and other common childhood illnesses.

Babies born via cesarean do not receive bacteria from the mother's gut, so an infant probiotic is recommended in these cases. Ensure you give your baby only an infant probiotic, as baby's have a different composition of bacteria (primarily bifidobacteria) in their intestines compared to that of adults. This is especially the case in breastfed babies.

Thrush

Pregnancy changes the acidity or pH of the vagina, which makes expectant mums more prone to developing thrush (or candida). Thrush is a yeast infection usually caused by a yeast-like fungus called Candida albicans.

Vaginal thrush usually produces a thick, white discharge that resembles curdled milk or cottage cheese, which can make this area very sore, red and itchy. The vaginal discharge of thrush usually has no odour, but it can make sex uncomfortable or painful and can cause a stinging sensation when urinating.

We all have fungus, bacteria and other microbes in our bodies. They are a normal part of our digestive systems. Good bacteria in our digestive tract usually keep these 'unfriendly microbes' in check. It is when there is an imbalance between the good and bad microbes in our body that there becomes a problem and we may develop conditions such as thrush.

Conditions that encourage thrush to flourish include antibiotic therapy, gestational diabetes, stress and a poor diet rich in processed, sugary foods.

Can thrush affect my baby?

It is important that pregnant women have a healthy balance of bowel bacteria during pregnancy and before the birth. When your baby comes down the birth canal it gulps vaginal fluids containing bacteria and other micro-organisms, which will 'set-up' the gut bacteria.

A newborn's gut is also inoculated by traces of the mother's faeces and from the surrounding environment. If the mother's bowel bacteria is unbalanced so too will her baby's.

Babies with unbalanced bowel bacteria are more prone to developing allergies such as eczema, asthma, hayfever and food intolerances in childhood. Taking a good probiotic supplement throughout pregnancy, especially in the last trimester of pregnancy, and while breastfeeding, can help reduce the risk of thrush and promote a healthy balance of bowel bacteria in the mother and baby. Babies born by c-section should take an infant probiotic after birth to help establish their gut flora.

Tips for preventing or treating thrush

- Avoid sugary foods. Fungus feeds off sugar!

- Avoid yeasty fermented foods such as yeast spreads (vegemite, marmite), yeast breads, mouldy cheeses, fermented vinegars, soya sauce, and miso. Also avoid mushrooms.

- Include natural probiotic-rich yoghurt in your diet and take a probiotic supplement daily. Check that your yoghurt is sugar-free.

- Eat garlic or take a garlic supplement as it has anti-fungal and immune boosting properties.

- Fresh coconut flesh contains caprilic acid, which is a powerful anti-fungal agent. Have it between meals or you could grate fresh coconut over natural yoghurt.

- Keep your genital area clean by using a gentle natural wash and water. Do not cleanse your vagina with douches, perfumed soaps or sprays, and avoid any antifungal treatments (oral, pessaries or creams) while pregnant and breastfeeding.

- Wash your clothes in a hypoallergenic, non-scented laundry detergent. Wear cotton underwear that will breathe. Avoid nylon underwear and synthetic tight leggings, stockings or pants, as they will create a warm environment for thrush to grow.

- If your partner has thrush he can re-infect you when having sex. He will need to be treated for thrush too. Abstaining from sex or wearing condoms until you are both thrush free is recommended. Signs that your partner has thrush include pain on urination and rough, dry red skin patches on his penis.

- Add either a cup of cider vinegar or a tablespoon of bicarbonate of soda into a bath. Or you could add 1 tablespoon of cider vinegar or baking soda to a cup of water and wash the area a few times a day.

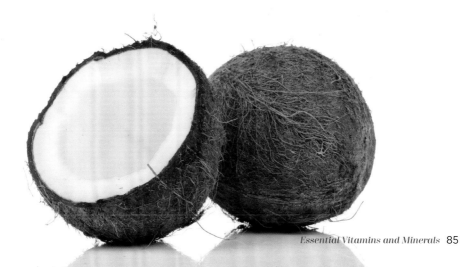

Fibre

- digestive health

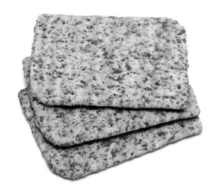

Dietary fibre helps keep our digestive tract in good working order and is also beneficial for strengthening our immune system and keeping cholesterol levels in check. Many pregnant women complain of constipation, so fibre is an important part of the daily diet to keep them regular and prevent the development of haemorrhoids. Fibre in foods also slows down the absorption of sugars into the blood stream, helping to keep blood sugar levels balanced.

High fibre foods include wholegrain cereals such as brown rice, quinoa, grainy breads, whole oats and oat bran, wheat germ, fruits, vegetables, and legumes. Psyllium husks are another easy way to get your bowels moving, try adding a heaped tablespoon to breakfast cereals or smoothies.

Always make sure you drink plenty of water whenever you increase your fibre intake to prevent digestive upsets.

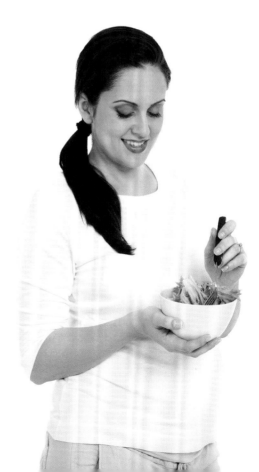

Constipation

Expectant mums often complain of constipation, especially during the early stages of pregnancy. One of the reasons pregnant women tend to suffer from constipation is due to increased progesterone, which is a pregnancy hormone that can slow your bowels down. Progesterone causes muscles throughout the body, including the digestive tract, to relax. As your growing uterus presses on your rectum, this can also make constipation worse. Not only does constipation make you feel uncomfortable, but constant straining can lead to haemorrhoids.

Tips for easing or preventing constipation

- One of the major causes of constipation is inadequate fluid intake and low-fibre intake, so make sure you drink plenty of water throughout the day and include plenty of fibre-rich foods in your diet. Fibre-rich foods include wholegrain cereals (whole oats, brown rice, quinoa) and grainy breads, fruits and vegetables, dried fruits and legumes. Wheat germ or psyllium husks can also be added to cereals or smoothies for extra fibre.

- Slippery elm powder is another effective, gentle fibre source that can help get things moving. Add a few teaspoons to water, juice, smoothies or mixed through yoghurt.

- Eating foods that have a natural, gentle laxative action can also be very helpful. Try snacking on some dried apricots, dates or prunes, or dice them up through muesli. You can also get prune and date spreads for toast, or prune juice.

- If you are supplementing with higher doses of iron this can also make you constipated. If this is the case ask your local naturopath or nutritionist for an iron supplement that won't cause constipation.

- Taking a probiotic supplement will help promote good bowel health and help relieve constipation.

- Getting regular exercise is important for easing constipation. Taking a walk, swim or prenatal yoga can really help.

- Do not use strong over the counter laxatives while you are pregnant. Some laxatives may cause harm to you and your baby, and could bring on uterine contractions.

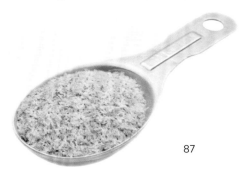

Stay well hydrated

Water is vital to good health, but is particularly important during pregnancy as your requirements increase. Expectant mums should make sure they stay well hydrated at all times by drinking at least 2 litres of water a day. You need plenty of water to flush toxins out of your kidneys and prevent urinary tract infections, as well as avoid constipation.

Keeping well hydrated will also support your dramatic increase in blood volume while pregnant. Water is needed for healthy blood production and flow, to carry important nutrients and oxygen to your growing baby. It's also needed to replenish the amniotic fluid, which surrounds and protects your baby, and women are advised to drink around a cup every hour.

Keeping well hydrated will also help prevent fluid retention and promote healthier skin. Women with severe morning sickness who are vomiting need to be careful not to become dehydrated. Sipping on water or an electrolyte drink, or sucking on homemade ice blocks will be beneficial.

Dehydration can stimulate contractions and can cause premature labour. It also causes a decrease in blood volume and therefore increases the concentration of oxytocin, the pregnancy hormone that causes uterine contractions.

It's a good idea to invest in a good water purifier or buy purified bottled water. Tap water can contain unwanted toxins such as pesticides, hormones, fluoride, and heavy metals, which you are trying to avoid during pregnancy.

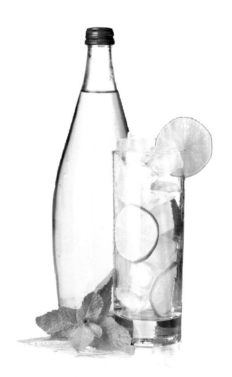

Carry a stainless steel or glass water bottle with you and sip throughout the day. If you find it hard to drink plain water add a splash of juice to give it some flavour. Caffeine-free herbal teas are delicious cold with some fresh lemon or mint.

Unhealthy fats

– what fats should I limit during pregnancy?

Fats are an important part of any pregnant woman's diet; however it needs to be the right type of fat. There are 3 main types of fats. The healthy mono and poly unsaturated fats, which include omega-3 essential fatty acids, are vital for your baby's brain and eye development. You find these good fats in oily fish, nuts, seeds and their oils, avocado, olive oil and wholegrain cereals.

Then you have saturated fats, which can cause high cholesterol levels and excessive weight gain if eaten too often. Being overweight while you are pregnant puts you at a greater risk of suffering from pregnancy complications such as hypertension, pre-eclampsia, gestational diabetes, and delivering a large baby. Having a diet high in saturated fats can also interfere with the body's metabolism of essential fatty acids (omega-3 fats). Small amounts of saturated fats are absolutely fine and are found mainly in animal based foods and full-fat dairy products.

The third type of fat is the bad one, trans-fats. These fats are artificially manufactured and formed when vegetable oils are heated at high temperatures.

Trans-fats are one of the main causes of heart disease and are linked to cancer. They cause good HDL cholesterol levels to drop and bad LDL cholesterol to rise.

Trans-fats are found in processed and fast foods, commercially baked goods, and some margarine. Small amounts of trans-fats can be found naturally in dairy and beef fat, but these natural fats have been found not to have the same detrimental effect on our health. You should try to avoid foods containing trans-fats. Look out for and avoid 'partially hydrogenated oil' or 'hydrogenated oil' on processed food labels.

Trans-fats offer no nutritional benefit to you or your baby. These harmful fats can cross the placental barrier so they should be avoided as much as possible. High intake of trans-fats has been linked to increased risk of pre-eclampsia. [8]

Some simple ways to switch to good fats

Do not use vegetable oils to cook with. The best oils to use for medium heat cooking like stir-fries include olive oil, grape seed and macadamia nut oils.

Oils that can be used for higher temperature cooking include safflower, sunflower, rice bran, coconut, and avocado oils.

Flaxseed oil is a good alternative to butter or margarine and is rich in healthy omega-3 fats - drizzle it over toast or salads but do not cook with it.

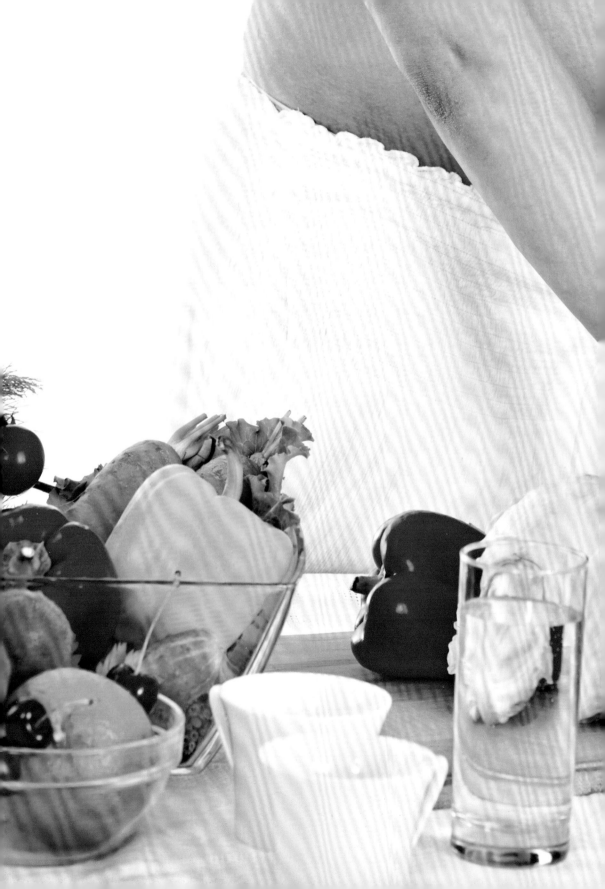

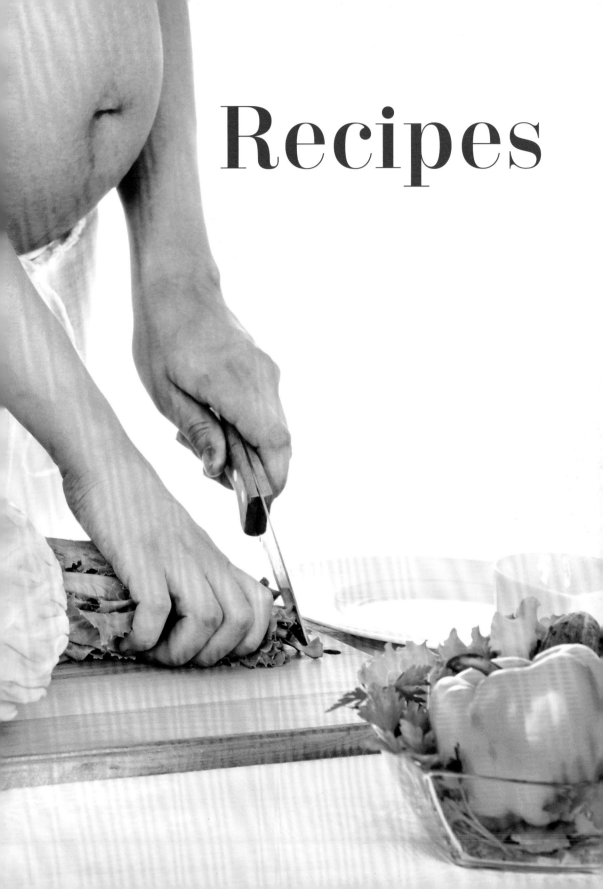

Recipes

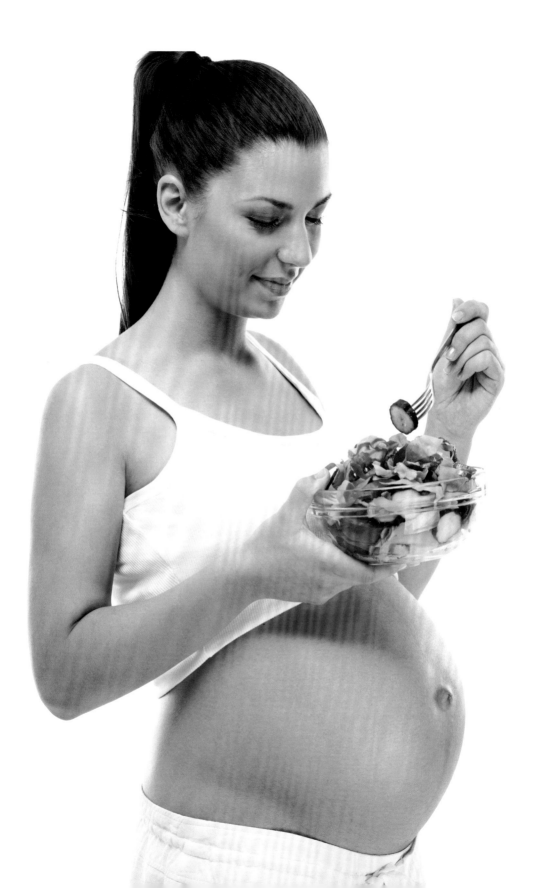

Breakfast

Berry Bircher Muesli

Super Breakie Booster

Quinoa Pear Porridge with Raspberries

Chia Seed Pudding

Mango Oat Porridge with Pomegranates

Green Kale Eggs

Nourishing Green Breakfast Bowl

Healthy Granola

Coconut Black Rice Porridge with Kefir

Snacks

Brazil Nut Oat Cookies

Ginger Glow Veggie Juice

Banana Berry Protein Smoothie

Super Trail Mix

Cashew Coconut Bliss Balls

Carrot Hummus with Roasted Pistachios

Green Goodness Smoothie

Super Veggie Juice

Gluten-free Lemony Chia Cakes

Protein Energy Squares

Lunch and Dinner

Salmon Kale Super Salad

Quinoa and Brown Rice Goji Salad

Zucchini Spaghetti Bolognaise

Salmon and Corn Kumera Patties

Roast Yams with Tahini Dressing

Spinach and Cauliflower Brown Rice Timbals

Lentil and Veggie Dahl with Quinoa

Beetroot and Coriander Super Salad

Dessert

Sugar-free Fruity Sorbet

Grilled Apricots with Raspberries

Raw Berry and Cashew Mini-Cheesecakes

Almond and Coconut Pancakes

Nectarine Pecan Crumble

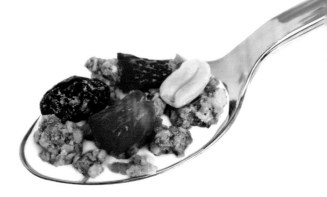

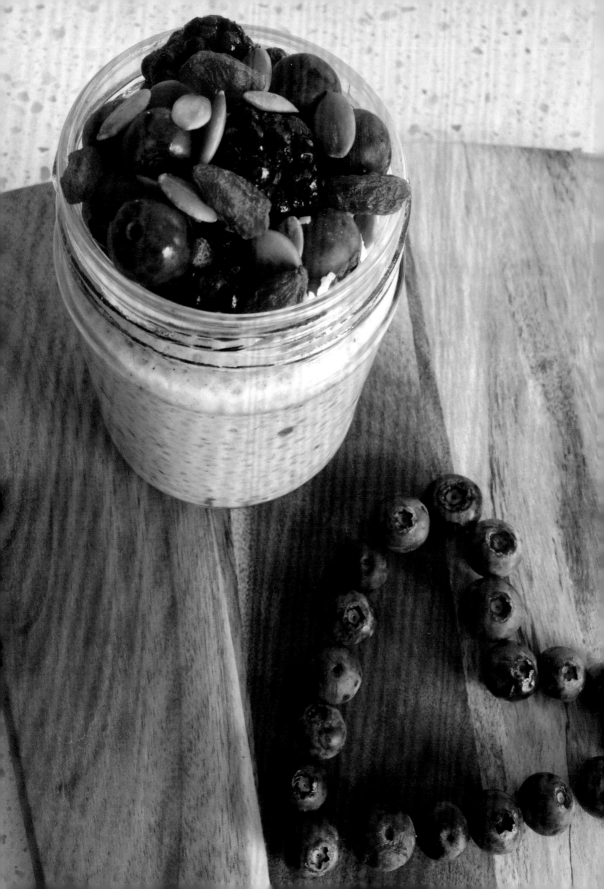

Breakfast

Berry Bircher Muesli

This Bircher muesli makes for a perfect, well-balanced breakfast. It is packed with fibre to help prevent constipation, as well as slow release complex carbohydrates and B vitamins to provide pregnant mums with a boost in energy. You will also get a good dose of antioxidants and probiotic goodness from this delicious breakfast.

Ingredients
1 cup rolled oats
1 tablespoon almond flakes
1 tablespoon sunflower or pumpkin seeds
1 tablespoon linseeds
1 ½ cups organic milk
½ cup organic natural yoghurt
1 grated apple or pear (leave skin on if using organic fruit)
½ cup mixed berries (strawberries, blueberries, mulberries and raspberries)

Method
Soak oats, nuts and seeds overnight in milk.

When ready to serve the next morning mix through yoghurt and fresh fruit.

Serves 2

Super Breakie Booster

Supercharge your breakfast with this super nut and seed mix. This is a fantastic way to give meals an extra nutritional boost, not to mention a lovely crunch. Raw nuts and seeds are jam-packed with a whole host of important nutrients needed in pregnancy including protein, zinc, magnesium, calcium, beneficial unsaturated fats and dietary fibre.

Ingredients
Choose from a variety of sunflower seeds, pumpkin seeds, chia seeds, flaxseeds, flaked almonds, crushed walnuts, activated buckinis (buckwheat seeds), sesame seeds and hemp seeds.

Method
Add 2 tablespoons of each of your chosen ingredients. Mix all ingredients together and store in a jar in the fridge. Add a big spoonful to breakfast cereals, smoothies, yoghurt, salads or fruit salads.

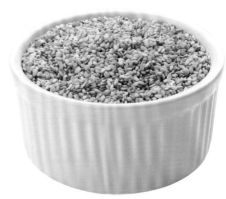

Quinoa Pear Porridge with Raspberries

Quinoa is a highly nutritious seed that's full of protein and fibre, and is a good source of iron and calcium, to help support mother and baby's health. This tasty breakfast is also rich in vitamin C and antioxidants, and it also has a low GI so it's perfect for keeping blood sugar levels stable and for reducing the risk of gestational diabetes.

Ingredients
1 cup of milk (almond, organic cow's, rice)
¾ cup quinoa flakes
1 pear, diced
1 tablespoon sunflower seeds
½ teaspoon ground cinnamon
Drizzle of raw honey (optional)
Organic yoghurt
Large handful of frozen or fresh raspberries
Handful of almonds

Method
Heat milk in a small saucepan, then add the quinoa. Cook for a few minutes, stirring often. Add in extra milk if you like a runnier porridge.

Add diced pear, seeds and cinnamon and then gently stir.

Take porridge off the heat and then stir in honey and yoghurt.

Serve topped with raspberries and some nuts or seeds.

Serves 1–2

Chia Seed Pudding

This gorgeous breakfast is incredibly nourishing for mother and baby. Chia seeds are a wonderful source of dietary fibre and an excellent way to prevent constipation during pregnancy. They also provide protein, calcium and beneficial omega-3 fats, which are all essential for your baby's brain and bone development. Coconut milk contains immune protective lauric and capric acid, as well as other fatty acids that are a superb energy source for mums and their growing babies.

Ingredients
3 tablespoons chia seeds
1 cup coconut milk (you can also use almond or cow's milk).
For extra sweetness you can add 1 teaspoon of raw honey, maple syrup, cinnamon, mashed banana or date paste.
Fruit for topping

Method
Place chia seeds and milk in a jar and leave in the fridge overnight.

In the morning top with your choice of fruits and nuts.

The chia pudding in the picture is served with a mango puree, figs, blueberries and walnuts.

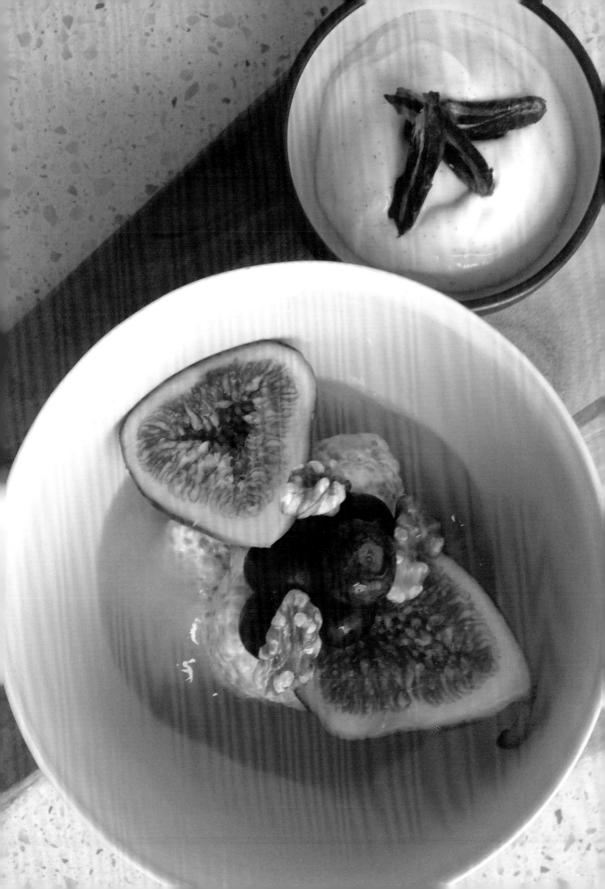

Mango Oat Porridge with Pomegranates

Oats are a fabulous source of slow release complex carbohydrates that will help keep blood sugar levels nice and balanced while providing energy for mum and for the baby's rapid growth. This delicious nourishing breakfast is also full of fibre to keep expectant mums regular, along with protein, vitamin C, zinc, calcium and probiotics. Pomegranates are a super fruit rich in potent antioxidants to help protect mother and baby.

Ingredients
¾ cup rolled oats
1 tablespoon pumpkin seeds
1 tablespoon sunflower seeds
1 ¾ cup milk (almond, rice, organic cow's)
1 mango (or banana)
Organic yoghurt
Pomegranate and berries for top

Method
Cook oats, seeds and milk in a saucepan for 5 minutes, until creamy.

Add mango and gently stir through.

Serve in a bowl topped with yoghurt, pomegranate and fresh berries.

Serves 2

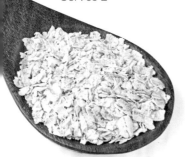

Green Kale Eggs

Kale is a super green 'leafie' vegetable that is rich in folate, an essential B vitamin for pregnant mothers. Kale also provides plenty of protective antioxidants, calcium, beta-carotene and vitamin K. Eggs are a fantastic protein source, and supply baby with choline and vitamin B12, which are vital for baby's brain and nervous system development.

Ingredients
½ bunch of kale
Cold pressed coconut oil
½ lemon
2 organic eggs
Pesto for topping
½ avocado
Handful of cherry tomatoes
Sesame seeds

Method
Wash kale well and remove stems.

Heat a little coconut oil in a fry pan and cook kale until it starts to soften. Then squeeze some lemon over the top.

Poach, boil or fry eggs, making sure they are cooked through.

Place kale on a plate, top with eggs, a spoonful of pesto, and serve with a side of avocado, cherry tomatoes and sesame seeds.

Serves 1

Nourishing Green Breakfast Bowl

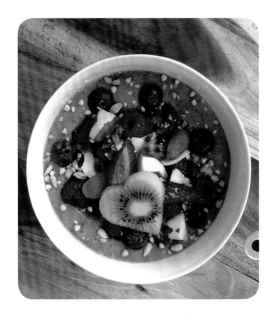

This delicious and healthy breakfast is a great way to increase your green leafy vegetables and folate levels. This important B vitamin is vital for pregnant mothers to reduce the risk of neural tube defects such as spina bifida. Spinach is a good source of vitamin B6 that can help ease fluid retention, which is common in pregnancy. You will also get plenty of vitamin C, nourishing 'good' fats, beta-carotene and protein from this breakfast.

Ingredients
2 tablespoons chia seeds
¼ cup raw nuts
1 cup baby spinach
1 cup coconut or almond milk
1 frozen banana
½ mango
½ avocado
1 teaspoon spirulina
Toppings: raw nuts, seeds, coconut flakes and fresh fruit

Method
Soak chia seeds in 4 tablespoons of water and let sit for 10 minutes until a gel forms.

Place nuts in food processor and blend until finely ground.

Add all the other ingredients, plus chia seed gel, and blend until a smooth consistency.

Top with raw nuts, seeds, coconut and fresh fruit.

Serves 1-2

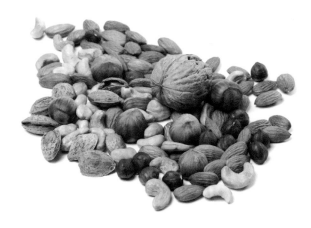

Healthy Granola

This delightful nutritious granola is an excellent way to start the day. Perfect served with a handful of fresh berries and almond milk, or with a good spoonful of organic natural yoghurt. This granola also makes a great topping for stewed fruit or yoghurt, for a healthy dessert or tasty snack.

Ingredients
3 tablespoons cold pressed coconut oil
¼ cup maple syrup or raw honey
1 teaspoon vanilla paste
3 cups rolled oats
½ cup pepitas and sunflower seeds
2 tablespoons sesame seeds
2 tablespoons flaxseeds
1 cup mixed raw nuts (Brazil, walnut, almonds, cashew)
1 cup coconut flakes
1 teaspoon ground cinnamon
½ cup dates, sliced
1 tablespoon goji berries

Method
Preheat oven to 180°C/350°F. Place grease-proof paper on an oven tray.

In a small saucepan on low heat melt coconut oil, maple syrup, and vanilla.

Place all other ingredients (except dried fruit) in a large bowl. Pour in coconut oil and gently combine.

Pour muesli mixture onto the oven tray and spread it out evenly.

Place in the oven for 30 minutes, tossing every 10 minutes.

Allow to cool and then add dates and goji berries. This muesli keeps well for a week in an airtight container in the refrigerator. You can also add some puffed brown rice, quinoa, buckwheat or millet for a lighter muesli.

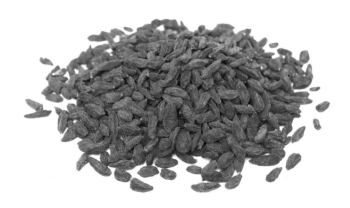

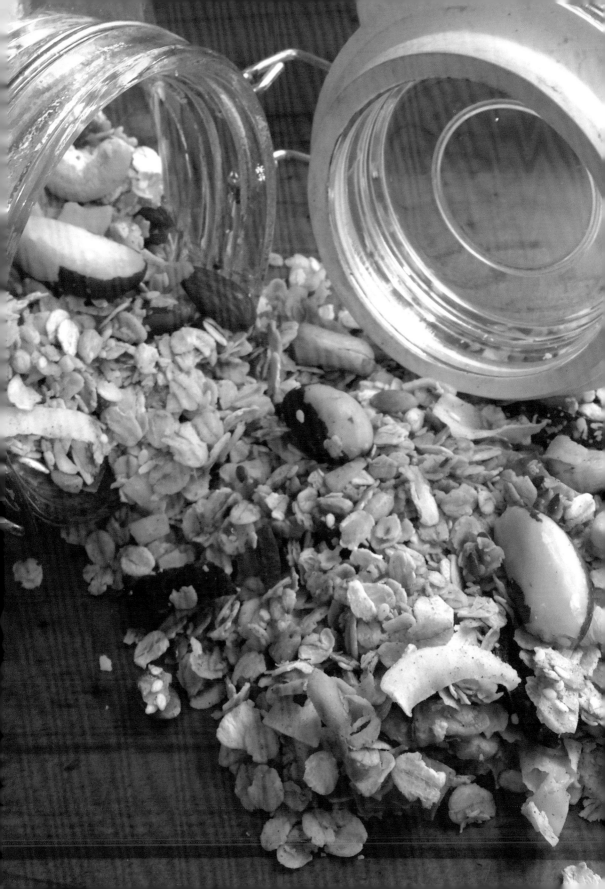

Coconut Black Rice Porridge with Kefir

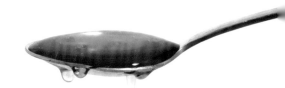

Black rice is considered a super food as it contains high levels of anthocyanin antioxidants, similar to those found in blueberries. Kefir gives this breakfast a probiotic boost to help support mother and baby's healthy immune function and reduce the risk of candida.

Ingredients
½ cup black rice
¾ cup water
½ teaspoon vanilla paste
½ can (200ml) coconut milk
1 teaspoon raw organic honey or maple syrup
Fruit, nuts, seeds and coconut flakes for topping
Kefir (coconut or dairy)

Method
Rinse rice well then add to a medium saucepan with the water, vanilla and coconut milk. Bring to the boil and then let simmer covered for 40 minutes, stirring often.

Transfer porridge to a bowl and top with desired fruit, nuts, seeds, coconut flakes and kefir.

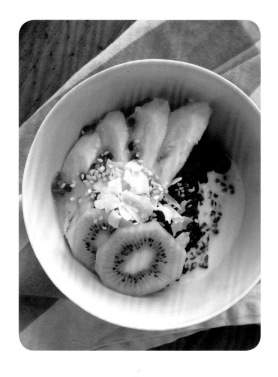

Snacks

Brazil Nut Oat Cookies

These scrumptious cookies make a nutritious snack or guilt-free after dinner treat. They are an excellent source of selenium, an important antioxidant mineral that plays a big role in supporting healthy thyroid and immune function. They are also rich in fibre, vitamin E and healthy fats, all required for a healthy pregnancy and baby.

Ingredients
1 ½ cups rolled oats
½ cup shredded dried coconut
½ cup Brazil nuts
2 tablespoons organic raw honey
2 ½ tablespoons cold pressed coconut oil
1 teaspoon vanilla essence
½ teaspoon ground cinnamon
1 tablespoon water

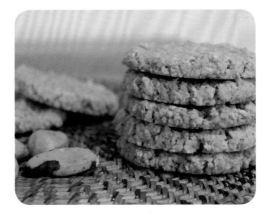

Method
Preheat your oven to 150°C/300°F.

Place oats, coconut and Brazil nuts in your food processor and pulse until well combined.

Add the honey, oil, vanilla essence and cinnamon, and mix until well combined. Then add the water and mix again.

Place spoonfuls of the cookie mixture on an oven tray lined with grease proof paper. Try using a tablespoon of mixture for each cookie. Flatten down your cookies and then pop them in the oven for around 35-40 minutes. Allow them to cool before eating.

Makes around 12 cookies

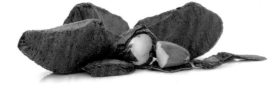

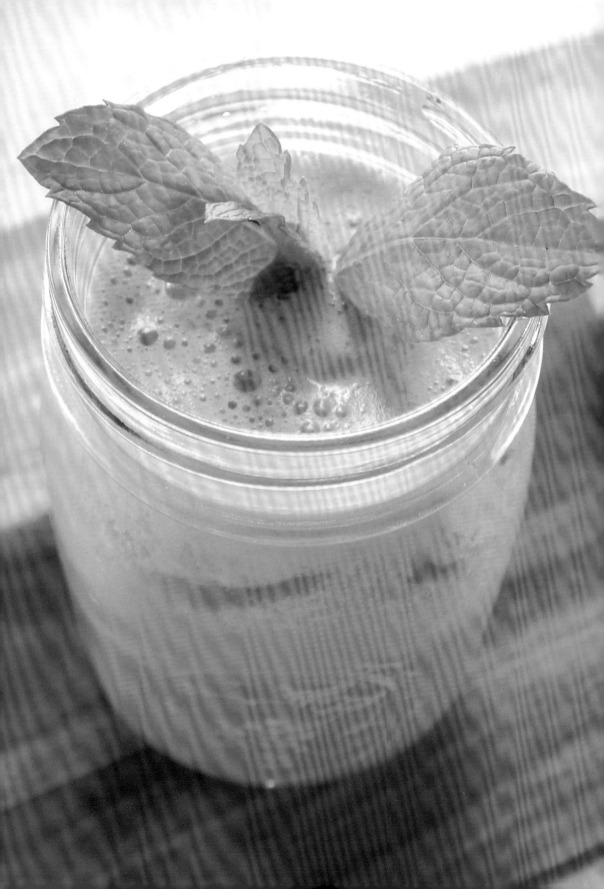

Ginger Glow Veggie Juice

This delicious juice with a ginger kick is a fantastic way to give your circulation and immune system a boost. This juice is ideal for helping ease morning sickness and is beneficial for fighting off colds and flu and other infections during pregnancy. You will also get a good dose of immune boosting beta-carotene, vitamin C and antioxidants in this gorgeous juice.

Ingredients
1 orange
2 celery sticks
2 medium carrots
Small slice of ginger
1 lime

Method
Juice ingredients, add some ice and enjoy.

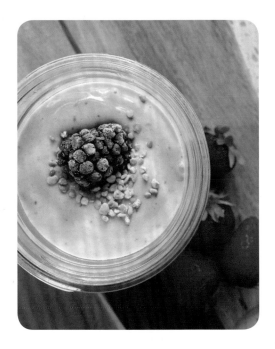

Banana Berry Protein Smoothie

This nutritious smoothie is packed with protein and super energy boosting ingredients. It makes a fantastic snack or breakfast on the go. This smoothie is loaded with protein to help meet women's increased need during pregnancy. It also provides plenty of calcium for a baby's bone growth, omega-3 fats for brain development and zinc, which is vital for a baby's health and for the prevention of stretch marks.

Ingredients
1 heaped tablespoon chia seeds
1 heaped tablespoon LSA (ground linseeds, sunflower seeds and almonds)
2 tablespoons brown rice protein powder
1 ½ cups almond milk
Handful of mixed berries
1 ripe frozen banana
2 tablespoons organic yoghurt or kefir
1 tablespoon cold pressed coconut oil
1 medjool date (remove seed)

Method
Place all ingredients in a blender and blend until well combined.

Makes 1-2 smoothies

Super Trail Mix

Trail mixes are the perfect protein rich snack to keep in your bag when you are out and about. A handful of trail mix will help keep your blood sugar levels balanced, which will stop you from snacking on unhealthy foods and will help reduce the risk of gestational diabetes. Dried fruits, especially dates, prunes and apricots act as a natural laxative, which will be beneficial for pregnant mums who are suffering from constipation.

Ingredients

Choose from a variety of raw and unsalted nuts and seeds – almonds, Brazil, hazelnuts, walnuts, cashews, sunflower seeds, pistachios and pepitas
Choose from a variety of dried fruits – apricots, goji berries, apple, dates, prunes, figs, banana, mango, cranberries and sultanas
Coconut flakes
Carob kibble or cacao nibs can also make a nice addition to trail mixes, for a chocolaty treat

Method

Add nuts, seeds, dried fruits, coconut and other ingredients into a large jar and store in the refrigerator.

Keep a jar at home or work and in your bag for when you get the munchies.

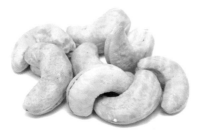

Cashew Coconut Bliss Balls

These moorish little balls are the perfect guilt-free snack. They are packed with protein to help keep blood sugar levels balanced and sugar cravings at bay. They contain plenty of zinc, which is essential for healthy immune function and a baby's growth and development, and nourishing healthy fats to support your baby's brain development. These balls are also a great way to help keep mums regular with their high fibre content.

Ingredients

1 cup raw cashews
1 cup coconut flakes
2 teaspoons vanilla paste
2 tablespoons flaxseeds
2 heaped tablespoons almond butter
10 medjool dates, remove seeds and roughly chop
Sesame seeds (to roll balls in)

Method

Place cashews, coconut, vanilla, flaxseeds and almond butter in your food processor and blend until well combined.

Add dates and blend well.

Roll mixture into balls and then roll in sesame seeds.

Place in the refrigerator in an airtight container.

Makes approximately 8 medium balls

Carrot Hummus with Roasted Pistachios

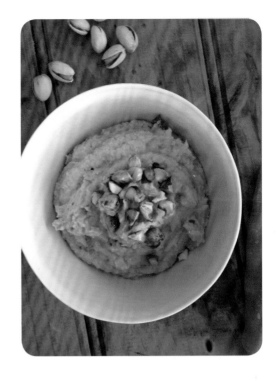

This super healthy dip is jam-packed with beta-carotene goodness to strengthen a mother and baby's immunity. Beta-carotene, which is converted to vitamin A in the body, plays an important role in your baby's eye development and vision. This tasty dip also provides plenty of protein, fibre and energy boosting B vitamins.

Ingredients
1 large carrot, peeled and diced
400g can of organic chickpeas, drained and rinsed
1 ½ tablespoon tahini
Juice of ½ lemon
1 garlic clove, crushed
2 tablespoons cold pressed olive oil
Pinch of sea salt
Handful of parsley
Handful of pistachios

Method
Steam carrots until they are cooked and then allow to cool.

Blend all ingredients except the pistachios in a food processor until it is nice and smooth.

Remove the shells from the pistachios and dry toast them in a pan. Transfer to a board and roughly chop.

Place the dip in a medium bowl and top with pistachios and a drizzle of olive oil.

Serve with celery and cucumber sticks, toasted flat breads or crackers.

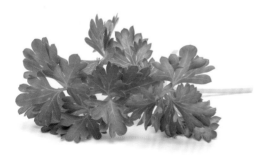

Green Goodness Smoothie

You will get a good dose of vitamin K from this wonderfully nourishing smoothie. Vitamin K is very important for pregnant women, as it is needed for blood clotting to help reduce the risk of excessive bleeding after birth. Your baby also needs a good supply of vitamin K to build strong and healthy bones. This juice is also bursting with antioxidants and beta-carotene, and the spirulina is a great source of iodine to support women's thyroid function during pregnancy and for a baby's optimal brain development.

Ingredients
1 cup ice cold water
3 cups chopped green leafies (use a variety of baby spinach, kale, swiss chard, lettuce and beet greens)
1 frozen banana
½ avocado
1 pear or apple
1 teaspoon spirulina
Juice of ½ lemon
1 tablespoon minced ginger (optional but great for easing morning sickness and boosting circulation)
2 teaspoons chia seeds

Method
Add all ingredients into your food processor and blend until well combined.

Makes 2 smoothies. Keep any leftovers in a jar in the refrigerator.

Super Veggie Juice

This beautiful juice combination is a great one for pregnant women as it contains high levels of protective antioxidants, beta-carotene and vitamin C. This juice can also help ease fluid retention, which is common in pregnancy, as celery acts as a natural diuretic. This juice is also a good source of potassium, another essential pregnancy nutrient to help keep blood pressure in check.

Ingredients
½ apple
½ large beetroot
1 carrot
1 celery stick
1 kale leaf
½ lemon

Method
Put all of the ingredients through your juicer.

Serve with ice and enjoy.

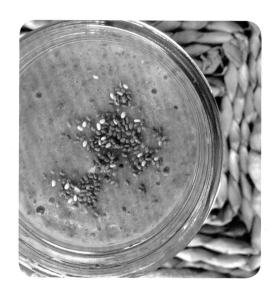

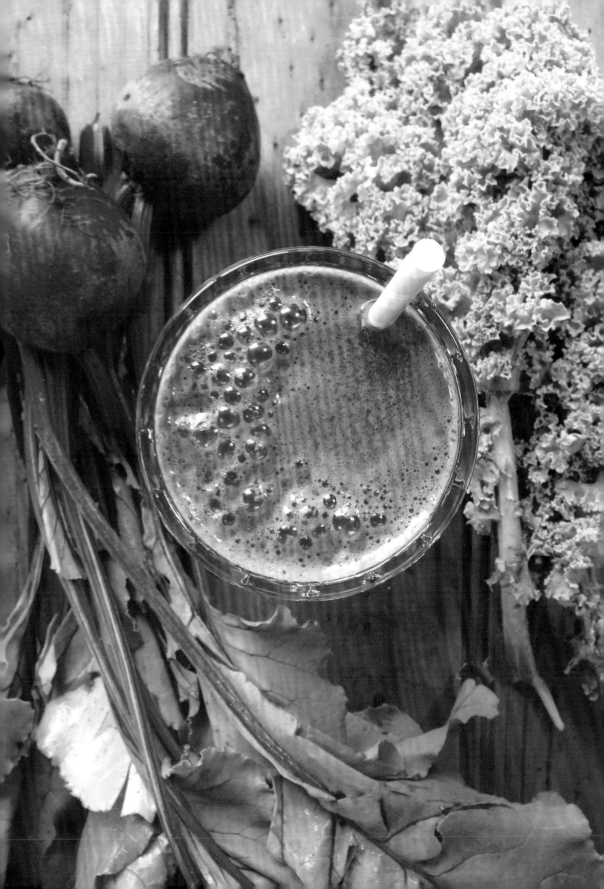

Gluten-free Lemony Chia Cakes

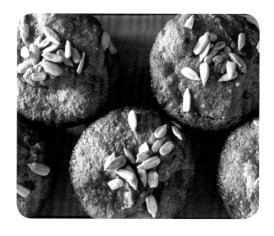

These delicious cakes make the perfect healthy treat with a cup of herbal tea. They contain plenty of protein to supply a baby with amino acids for optimal growth, healthy fats for brain development, and calcium for strong bones. These cakes also provide zinc, which is beneficial for mothers to prevent stretch marks.

Ingredients
1 ½ cups almond flour
¼ cup chia seed meal
1 ½ tablespoon gluten-free baking powder
½ cup raw honey or maple syrup
4 organic eggs
⅓ cup coconut oil, melted
¼ cup natural yoghurt
1 tablespoon organic lemon rind
2 tablespoons sunflower seeds, for top

Topping
1 tablespoon raw honey or maple syrup
1 tablespoon organic lemon juice

Method
Preheat oven at 160°C/320°F.

Place paper muffin cups in a 12 hole muffin tray.

Place all ingredients except the sunflower seeds in your food processer and blend until well combined.

Pour mixture into cupcake holes and sprinkle with sunflower seeds.

Bake for 30 minutes or until skewer comes out cleanly from the centre.

Mix extra honey and lemon together. Pour 1 teaspoon over each cake while still hot.

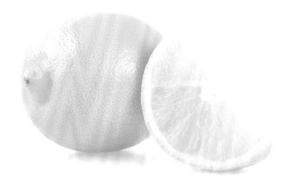

Protein Energy Squares

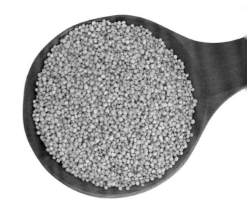

If you're looking for a nutritious protein-rich snack to keep you going until your next meal, these tasty little squares are just what you need. They're loaded with protein and fibre and contain plenty of beneficial fats that are essential for a baby's brain function and development.

Ingredients

¼ cup pumpkin seeds
¼ cup sunflower seeds
2 heaped tablespoons chia seeds
¾ cup desiccated coconut
½ cup puffed brown rice or puffed quinoa
¼ cup raw cashews or almonds
16 Medjool dates, remove seeds and roughly chop
2 heaped tablespoons tahini

Method

Pulse all dry ingredients in your food processor until ground. Transfer to a bowl.

Place dates and tahini into the food processor and blend until it forms a paste. Add dry ingredients and pulse until well combined.

Use your hands to press the mixture into individual squares and top with a whole almond and some pumpkin seeds.

Store in the refrigerator in an airtight container.

Makes around 12-14 squares

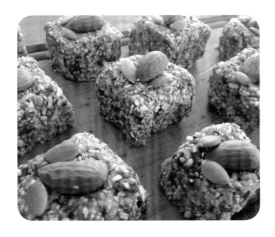

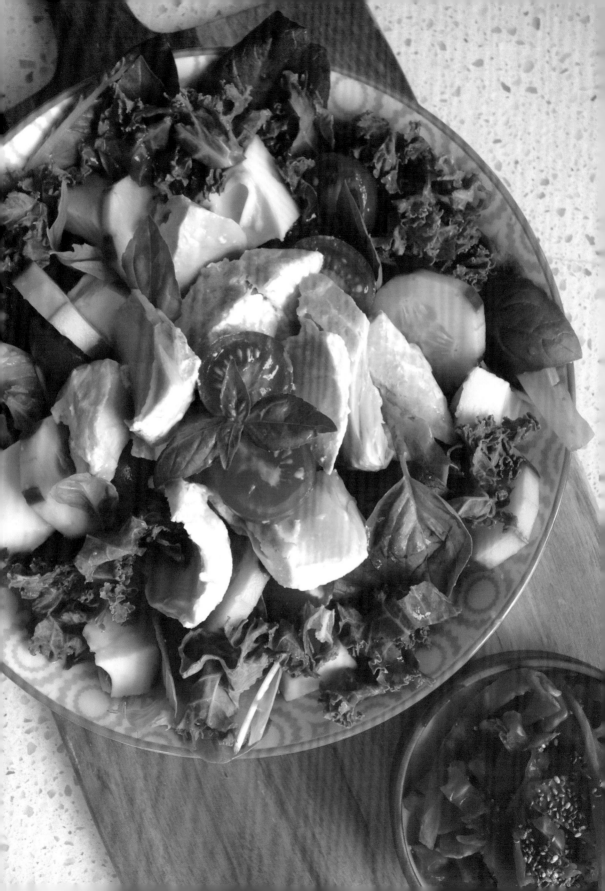

Lunch and Dinner

Salmon Kale Super Salad

Salmon is one of the best sources of healthy omega-3 fats, which growing babies need for healthy brain and nervous system development. Mothers also need a good supply of this healthy fat to keep their skin supple, more elastic and less prone to stretch marks. Kale is one of the healthiest green leafy vegetables around. It will deliver plenty of vitamin K and antioxidants, along with some extra omega-3. Like other brassica veggies, eating kale regularly will help support proper liver detoxification.

Ingredients
Juice of ½ lemon
1 tablespoon cold pressed flaxseed or olive oil
½ teaspoon raw honey
Pinch of sea salt
2 kale leaves, remove stems and finely chop leaves
1 small salmon fillet
A big handful of mixed green leaves (baby spinach, rocket, watercress, parsley)
Handful of cherry tomatoes
½ small avocado
1 tablespoon pumpkin seeds

Method
Mix lemon juice, oil, honey and sea salt together. Place kale in a bowl and pour lemon dressing over it, gently massaging it into the kale to soften it.

Grill or oven bake salmon and then break into large pieces.

Place kale and green leaves in a serving bowl and top with tomato, avocado, pumpkin seeds and salmon.

To give this dish a probiotic boost serve with a side of fermented vegetables like sauerkraut. This is a great way to promote a healthy balance of bowel flora for mother and baby.

Serves 1-2

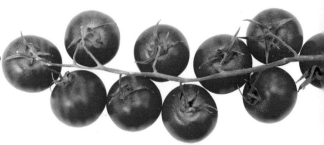

Quinoa and Brown Rice Goji Salad

This hearty salad is jam-packed with super healthy ingredients to support a healthy pregnancy and growth of your little one, including protein, fibre, iron, vitamin C and zinc. Goji berries are celebrated as a super food due to their high levels of protective antioxidants. This salad is delicious served cold or warm.

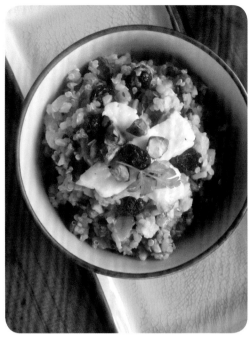

Ingredients
1 cup quinoa, rinsed well
1 cup brown rice, rinsed well
⅓ cup goji berries
1 organic orange, juiced and zested
1 onion, thinly sliced
½ cauliflower or broccoli, cut into small pieces
¾ cup almonds, roughly chopped
1 cup fresh mint, roughly chopped
1 cup fresh coriander, roughly chopped

Dressing
Juice of 1 lemon
1 clove garlic, crushed
¼ cup cold pressed flaxseed or olive oil
Pinch of sea salt

Method
Cook quinoa in a saucepan with a little olive oil for 1 minute, then pour in 2 cups of water. Bring to the boil and simmer with the lid on for 15 minutes. Allow to sit for 5 minutes.

Cook brown rice in a separate saucepan for around 40 minutes, until tender.

Soak goji berries in orange juice with zest.

Cook onion in frying pan with some olive oil for around 8-10 minutes then set aside. Cook cauliflower in fry pan until cooked through.

In a large bowl add cauliflower, onion, rice, quinoa, goji berries (with the orange juice and zest), nuts and fresh herbs.
To make the dressing whisk lemon juice, garlic, olive oil and sea salt. Pour dressing over salad and gently toss.

Serves 4-6

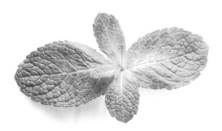

Zucchini Spaghetti Bolognaise

This dish is a light and lovely take on an old favourite. You will get plenty of important pregnancy nutrients from this delicious meal including high levels of iron, folate, protein, beta-carotene and zinc. Ideal for coeliacs or anyone with a gluten-intolerance.

Ingredients
6 large zucchinis
1 onion, finely sliced
400g organic lamb mince
1 garlic clove, crushed
1 carrot, grated
1 celery stick, finely sliced
½ red capsicum
2 x 400g cans organic tomatoes
2 heaped tablespoons tomato paste
Small handful of fresh basil, finely chopped
3 tablespoons pesto
Grated cheese to serve

Method
Using a julienne peeler (or spiral slicer) peel zucchinis into long spaghetti strips.

Cook onion and lamb in a pan on medium heat with a little olive oil until cooked through. Add garlic and vegetables and cook until they start to soften. Pour in tomatoes, paste and basil. Turn down the heat and allow to simmer until sauce reduces and vegetables are cooked through.

To make your spaghetti, heat a little olive oil in a pan and add zucchini strips. Gently toss with pesto for 2-3 minutes until zucchini starts to soften.

Plate up zucchini, top with bolognaise sauce and some grated cheese, and serve with a big green salad.

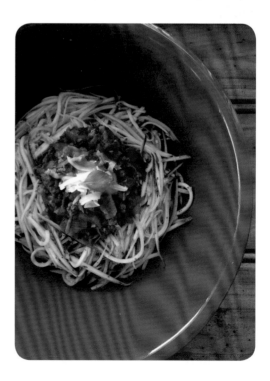

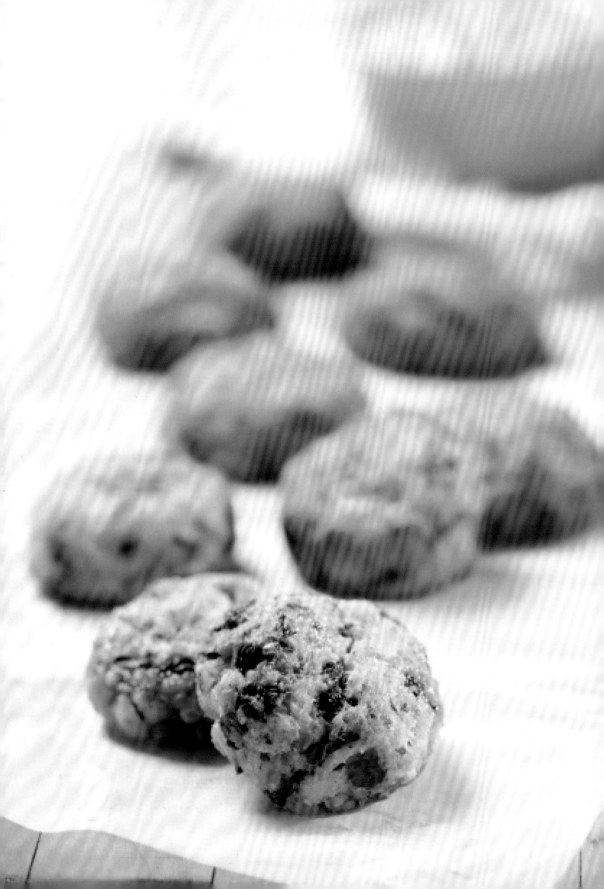

Salmon and Corn Kumera Patties

Packed with protein and omega-3 goodness, these salmon patties make the perfect snack, nutritious meal served with salad or vegetables, or healthy burger on a wholemeal roll.

Ingredients

500g kumera (orange sweet potato)
415g can salmon, drained
½ red onion, finely chopped
¼ cup fresh basil, chopped
¾ cup corn kernels
1 small garlic clove, crushed

Method

Cut kumera into pieces and steam for around 10 minutes until cooked through. Mash kumera in a bowl, add salmon, onion, basil, a pinch of salt and pepper, corn kernels and the garlic clove.

Gently combine ingredients, divide into small patties and cook in a frying pan with a little olive oil, or cook in the oven on 190°C/370°F for around 20 minutes.

Serve with a handful of baby spinach, slices of avocado, and a spoonful of tzatziki, mango or tomato chutney.

Makes approximately 12

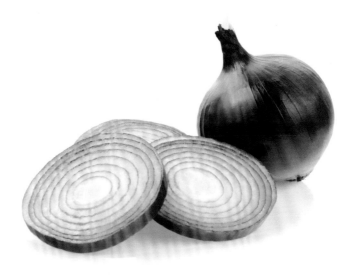

Roast Yams with Tahini Dressing

This delightfully earthy dish contains plenty of vital pregnancy nutrients. Tahini is an excellent source of calcium and protein to support a baby's growing bones. Yams are rich in slow release complex carbohydrates to provide extra energy for your rapidly growing baby, without sending your blood sugar and insulin levels soaring.

Ingredients
2 large yams or sweet potatoes, use a variety of colours if you can
Cold pressed olive oil

Dressing
⅓ cup tahini
⅓ cup water
¼ cup lemon juice
2 garlic cloves, crushed
Pinch of sea salt
1 teaspoon raw organic honey or maple syrup

Method
Preheat oven to 200°C/390°F and line a baking tray with baking paper.

Cut yams into large chunks and leave skin on if you are using organic produce. Steam yams until they are par cooked. Place yams on baking tray and drizzle with olive oil then place in the oven for around 40 minutes.

Place all of the dressing ingredients in your food processor and blend until you have a smooth consistency.

Drizzle dressing over yams and enjoy. This dressing also makes a lovely salad dressing so store any leftovers in a jar in the refrigerator.

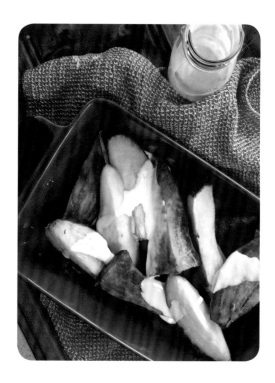

Spinach and Cauliflower Brown Rice Timbals

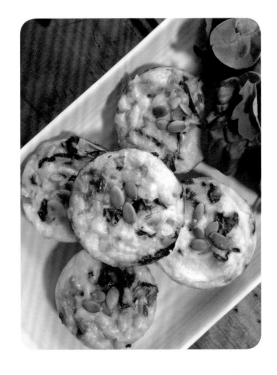

These tasty rice timbals make an excellent protein rich snack or main meal served with a big green salad. They are a great way for pregnant women to increase their folate levels, as well as their calcium and protein intake. Eggs are one of the best food sources of vitamin D, which is important for a baby's bone development. This dish is delicious served hot or cold the next day for lunch.

Ingredients
1 cup cauliflower, diced small
½ cup corn kernels
1-2 garlic cloves, crushed
1 ½ cups spinach, finely chopped
Cold pressed coconut oil
1 cup cooked brown rice
6 organic eggs
⅓ cup milk
⅓ cup grated cheddar cheese
Pumpkin seeds for top

Method
Preheat oven to 200°C/390°F and grease a 12-hole muffin tray with a little coconut oil.

Stir fry cauliflower, corn, garlic and spinach in a pan with some coconut oil until cooked through. Then stir through cooked brown rice.

In a medium bowl, whisk eggs and milk and then stir through cheese.

Divide cauliflower and rice mixture up evenly into muffin holes, then pour egg mixture over the top of each.

Top with pumpkin seeds and cook in the oven for 30-35 minutes until timbals are cooked through and a skewer comes out of the centre cleanly.

Makes 12

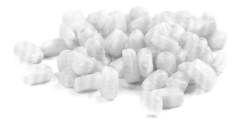

Lentil and Veggie Dahl with Quinoa

This tasty Indian dish is a quick and highly nutritious meal. Lentils are an excellent source of iron, which is essential for pregnant women to support extra red blood cell production and the delivery of oxygen and nutrients to their growing baby. This dish also supplies plenty of protein, fibre, B vitamins and zinc, which are all essential nutrients for a mother and her baby. This dahl goes beautifully with warm wholemeal pita bread, tzatziki, brown rice or quinoa.

Ingredients

1 cup quinoa, rinsed well (white, golden, red or black)
1 cup red lentils, rinsed well
2 teaspoons finely grated fresh ginger
1 small onion, finely chopped
1-2 garlic cloves, crushed
1 carrot, diced
Handful of diced cauliflower or broccoli
1 celery stalk, sliced
½ cup peas (fresh or frozen)
2 teaspoons ground turmeric
1 teaspoon garam masala
1 teaspoon ground coriander
1 x 400g can tomatoes
Small handful of fresh coriander, chopped

Method

Heat some coconut oil in a saucepan, add quinoa and cook for around a minute. Slowly add enough water to cover the quinoa and a pinch of sea salt and bring to the boil. Reduce the heat and let it simmer covered for 15 minutes. Turn the heat off and allow quinoa to sit with the lid on for another 5 minutes.

While the quinoa is cooking, in another saucepan place lentils with 3 cups of cold water. Bring to the boil, then reduce heat and simmer for around 10-12 minutes, stirring regularly, until lentils are cooked through.

Add a little coconut oil to a fry pan and cook ginger, onion and garlic until tender. Add carrot, cauliflower, celery, peas and spices, and stir-fry until they are cooked through.

Add tomatoes to the vegetable mix, along with lentils and fresh coriander and cook for another few minutes.

Serve topped with quinoa, some fresh herbs and seeds.

Serves 4

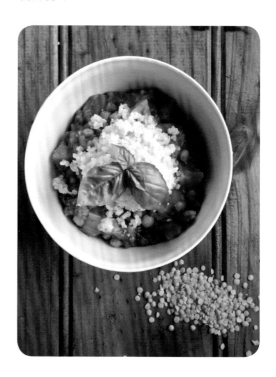

Beetroot and Coriander Super Salad

This fabulous antioxidant rich salad will offer you and your baby protection from oxidative stress along with helping bolster your immunity. It only takes minutes to whip up and it's delicious on its own, served with fish or chicken, or as a healthy sandwich filler.

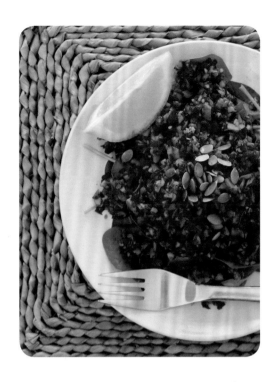

Ingredients
1 large carrot
1 small beetroot
A good handful of fresh coriander
1 celery stick
1 apple
A small piece of ginger
1 lemon
A handful of baby spinach leaves
A handful of pumpkin seeds

Method
Roughly chop carrot, beetroot, coriander, celery, apple and ginger and put in your food processor. Pulse until you have a finely chopped salad.

Toss lemon juice through salad and then serve on a bed of baby spinach, topped with pumpkin seeds.

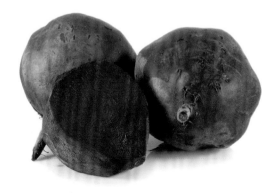

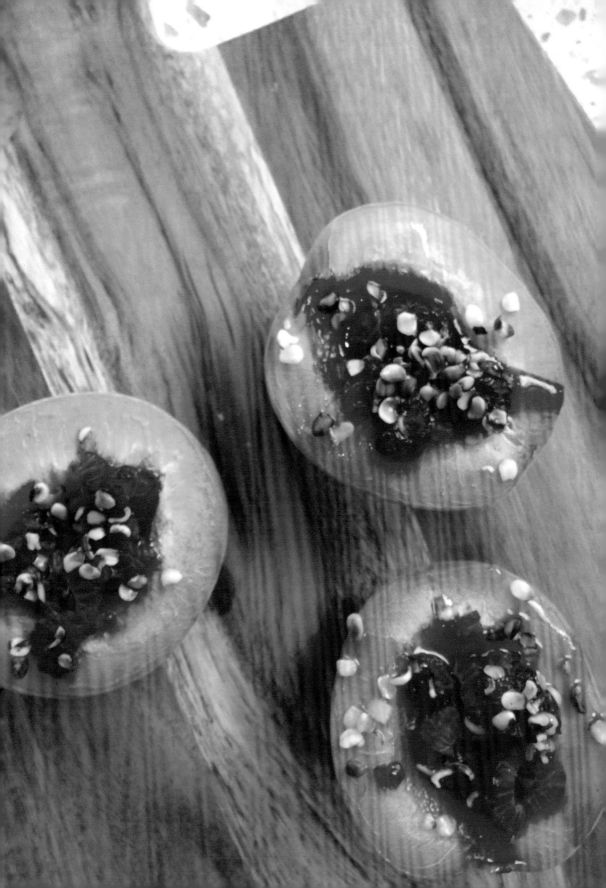

Desserts

Sugar-free Fruity Sorbet

Now you can have all the pleasure of sorbet without all the sugar. This lovely refreshing dessert can be very soothing for women suffering from morning sickness and it is bursting with antioxidants, vitamin C and beta-carotene.

Ingredients
Choose from a variety of fruits: watermelon, pineapple, kiwi, raspberries, strawberries, banana, or mango.

Method
Roughly chop fruit and place in a container in the freezer for a few hours or overnight. Place frozen fruit in your food processor and blend until you have a soft sorbet consistency.

Serve immediately.

Leftovers can be put back in the freezer.

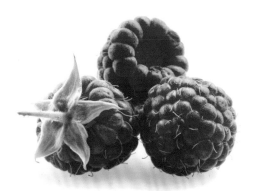

Grilled Apricots with Raspberries

This simple yet delightful healthy dessert is full of beta-carotene goodness to assist with your baby's healthy eye development and vision. Yoghurt is an excellent source of protein, calcium and beneficial bacteria to help support both mother and baby's health.

Ingredients
4 fresh apricots
Raspberries (frozen or fresh) for topping
Seeds (flax, sesame, chia, or hemp)
Raw honey
Organic natural yoghurt

Method
Cut apricots in half and top with raspberries and seeds.

Drizzle on a little honey.

Place under the griller for 5 minutes. Serve with yoghurt.

Leftovers are delicious the next day eaten with muesli and yoghurt.

Raw Berry and Cashew Mini Cheesecakes

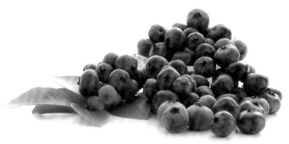

These gorgeous little cheesecakes are almost too good to be true. They not only taste amazing but they are full of pregnancy friendly nutrients like protein, calcium, fibre, zinc, magnesium and vitamin C.

Ingredients
1 cup almond meal
¼ cup shredded coconut
¾ cup Medjool dates, remove seeds
2 cups raw cashew nuts (soak for an hour)
¼ cup maple syrup or raw honey
Juice of 1 ½ lemons
2 teaspoons vanilla extract or paste
Blueberries and raspberries for top

Method
To make the crust, place almond meal, coconut and dates in your food processor and pulse until well combined and the mixture starts to stick together.

Divide and press mixture evenly into 12-muffin tin holes.

To make the filling blend soaked cashews, maple syrup, lemon juice and vanilla until smooth.

Pour evenly over bases in muffin tin and top with berries. Place cheesecakes in the freezer for a couple of hours to set.

Take cheesecakes out of the freezer to defrost a little before serving.

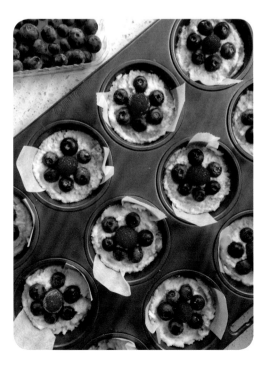

Almond and Coconut Pancakes

These light and fluffy gluten-free pancakes make a lovely dessert or snack served with fresh fruit and yoghurt. These pancakes will supply you and your baby with a good dose of protein and calcium, to help support a baby's bone growth; healthy fats, which are essential for their nervous system development; and zinc to help fight off infections. You will also get plenty fibre in this dessert to help keep you nice and regular.

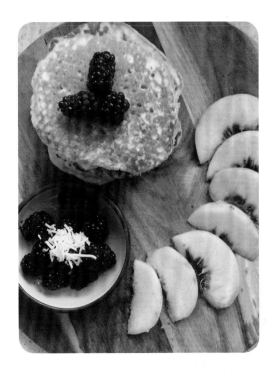

Ingredients
1 ½ cups almond flour
2 tablespoons coconut flour
¼ teaspoon salt
¾ teaspoon baking soda
6 organic eggs
¼ cup milk
2 tablespoons honey or maple syrup
1 tablespoon coconut oil
Fruit and organic yoghurt for topping

Method
Mix dry ingredients together in a large bowl.

In another bowl, whisk eggs, milk, honey and oil together.

Pour wet ingredients into the dry ingredients and mix until well combined and smooth.

Heat a little coconut oil in a frying pan over a medium heat. Pour spoonfuls of mixture into the pan and cook for 3 minutes (or until pancakes starts to bubble), flip and then cook on the other side for 3 minutes.

Serve with sliced fruit and yoghurt.

Makes approximately 14 medium pancakes

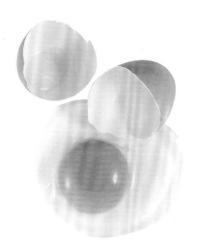

Nectarine Pecan Crumble

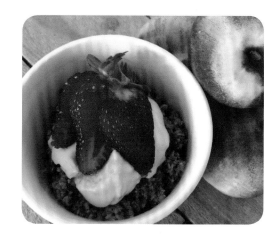

Nectarines are loaded with vitamin C and beta-carotene, which are two super important nutrients needed for a strong and functioning immune system, and for collagen production. Brazil nuts are packed with protein and healthy fats, and they're one of the best sources of selenium around, which is an important antioxidant mineral helping to support healthy thyroid function. Pepitas are a great way to boost your zinc levels along with supporting healthy immune function and healing after the birth.

Ingredients
½ cup rolled oats
½ cup shredded coconut
10 Brazil nuts
3 tablespoons pepitas (pumpkin seeds)
2 tablespoons raw honey or maple syrup
5 nectarines (or peaches or pears)
Organic vanilla yoghurt and strawberries for top

Method
Place oats, coconut, Brazil nuts and pepitas in your food processer and blend well. Pour into a small bowl.

Add honey to oat mixture and combine well.

Peel and cut nectarines and place in 4 ramekin dishes, then top with crumble mixture.

Place in a 200°C/390°F oven for 10 minutes.

Top with a spoonful of vanilla yoghurt and a strawberry to serve.

Makes 4 individual crumbles

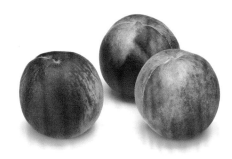

References

1. Maryse F. Bourchard, Jonathan Chevrier, Kim G. Harley, Katherine Kogut, Michelle Vedar, Norma Calderon, Celina Trujillo, et al. Prenatal Exposure to Organophosphate Pesticides and IQ in 7-Year-Old Children. Environmental Health Perspectives, 119(8), Aug 2011.

2. Francois CA, Connor SL, Wander RC, Connor WE. Acute effects of dietary fatty acids on the fatty acids of human milk. American Journal of Clinical Nutrition 1998; 67:301-308.

3. Petra Rattue. "Mothers Who Eat Fish While Pregnant Produce Offspring With Better Cognitive Development." Medical News Today. MediLexicon, Intl., 1 Feb. 2012. Web. 30 Apr. 2012. http://www.medicalnewstoday.com/articles/241045.php.

4. Yale School of Medicine. The FASEB Journal. Hormones and Cancer. Vol. 24, Issue 3. March 2010.

5. Hiten D. Mistry and Paula J. Williams. The Importance of Antioxidant Micronutrients in Pregnancy, Review Article. Oxidative Medicine and Cellular Longevity Volume 2011 (2011), Article ID 841749, 12 pages.

6. Sarbattama Sen, Rebecca A. Simmons, "Maternal Antioxidant Supplementation Prevents Adiposity in the Offspring of Western Diet-Fed Rats," Diabetes, Dec. 2010.

7. Samuli Rautava, Marko Kalliomaki, Erika Isolauri. Probiotics during pregnancy and breast-feeding might confer immunomodulatory protection against atopic disease in the infant. Journal of Allergy and Clinical Immunology, 2002;109:119-21.

8. Williams MA, King IB, Sorensen TK, et al. Risk of preeclampsia in relation to elaidic acid (trans fatty acid) in maternal erythrocytes. Gynecologic and Obstetric Investigation 1998;46:84-7.

Index